Functional Training
Everyone's Guide to the New Fitness Revolution

ROSEMARIE GIONTA ALFIERI

FOREWORD BY
PAUL CHEK

PREFACE BY
VERN GAMBETTA

PHOTOGRAPHS BY
PETER FIELD PECK

HATHERLEIGH PRESS
NEW YORK

A GETFITNOW.COM BOOK

Functional Training–Everyone's Guide to the New Fitness Revolution
A Getfitnow.com Book®

© Copyright 2001 RoseMarie Gionta Alfieri

Getfitnow.com is a registered trademark of The Hatherleigh Company, Ltd.

Hatherleigh Press/Getfitnow.com Books
An Affiliate of W.W. Norton and Company, Inc.
5-22 46th Avenue, Suite 200
Long Island City, NY 11101
Toll Free 1-800-528-2550
Visit our websites getfitnow.com and hatherleighpress.com

Disclaimer:
Before beginning any exercise program consult your physician. The author and the publisher disclaim any liability, personal or professional, resulting from the application or misapplication of any of the information in this publication.

Hatherleigh Press/Getfitnow.com books are available for bulk purchase, special promotions and premiums. For more information on reselling and special purchase opportunities, please call us at 1-800-528-2550 and ask for the Special Sales Manager.

Library of Congress Cataloging-in-Publication Data

Alfieri, RoseMarie.
   Functional training : everyone's guide to the new fitness revolution /
   researched and written by RoseMarie Alfieri ; introduction by Paul Chek ;
   foreword by Vern Gambetta ; photographs by Peter Field Peck.
       p. cm.
   Includes bibliographical references.
   ISBN 1-57826-063-9 (alk. paper)
   1. Physical fitness. 2. Exercise. 3. Health. I. Title.

RA781 .A54 2001
613.7—dc21

2001024976

Layout and Design by Fatema Tarzi

Text Photos by Peter Field Peck

VISIT THE AUTHOR ON THE INTERNET AT
www.getfitnow.com

10 9 8 7 6 5 4 3 2 1
Printed in Canada on acid-free paper.

— TABLE OF CONTENTS —

— DEDICATIONS —

This book is dedicated to my husband Michael in gratitude for his unfailing support, love and generosity; and to my parents, Camillo and Gloria, for their loving guidance throughout the years.

— ACKNOWLEDGEMENTS —

Much thanks to my publishers, Andrew Flach and Kevin Moran, at Hatherleigh Press for their support and vision for this book.

Thanks also to Susan Grzybowski, fitness trainer and group instructor for The New York Health and Racquet Club, who was a most gracious and professional model.

To Matt Bloom, our male model, for his good humor and patience during a long day of shooting.

To the technical assistance and support that James Villepigue provided during our shoot.

Finally, a special thanks to the following experts who, despite hectic schedules, gave of their time and knowledge as contributors to this book: Paul Chek, Christine (CC) Cunningham, Paul Frediani, Vern Gambetta, Michael Jenniex, and Annette Lang.

— FOREWORD —
THE FUNCTIONAL EXERCISE ERA
by Paul Chek

I have been involved in sports conditioning since I began wrestling in the third grade and got my first chance to see what can happen to one's body when over-exposed to traditional isolation, or machine-based training, while I was a member and trainer of the U.S. Army Boxing Team at Ft. Bragg, North Carolina in 1984. To get on the boxing team, all anyone had to do was schedule an appointment for a tryout and if you could beat any of the three current members in any given weight class, you were awarded his position on the team. Tryouts were always interesting and always stressful!

Quite often, the door to the boxing gym would swing open in the middle of our long, grueling practices and in would walk a poor unsuspecting soldier who was obviously into bodybuilding. As soon as we saw "that puffed up tight look" that is so common to those that utilize isolation training as their primary form of conditioning, we always felt a quiet sense of relief. Just to make a point, Coach Johnson or Coach Smith would throw the bodybuilder types in the ring with someone two, or even three weight classes below their weight. Regardless of the fact that they were fighting against men far smaller and less powerful than they would fight in a real boxing tournament, the bodybuilder types seldom lasted past the second round. Truthfully, quite often the first round was enough to see the towel come flying into the ring, signaling that the person trying out was dangerously close to being knocked out and could not adequately protect himself!

Although watching bodybuilders get manhandled in the ring by men much smaller than them was entertaining, it certainly created a challenging situation for me as the trainer. I had been lifting free weights since I was twelve years old and had found it to be beneficial in all the sports I played, including boxing. It was well known among team members and coaches that I had one punch knockout power, yet they resisted my inclusion of more than a very small amount of weight training in the program for fear that "it would slow the fighters down." This fear was repeatedly driven by seeing how bodybuilders, or boxers-turned-bodybuilders, performed in the ring during tryouts.

To minimize the coaches' and fighters' fear of becoming slow, I had to play a little game with their minds; I used weighted chin-ups, push-ups and cable exercises as the primary form of resistance training. At the end of the training day, two to three days a week depending on how heavy the fight schedule was, we would finish with circuit training that included free weights, machines, cables, medicine ball work and calisthenics. Performing exercises like biceps curls, triceps push downs, or any such isolation exercise was almost like asking the coach if we could all have an ice cream Sunday, the night before a fight! There was no way he would have let us do either! Using this type of training, I was able to keep the coaches happy and keep the boxers strong. I helped build knockout power in the fighters using exercises that are classically referred to as integration or compound exercises (multiple muscles and joints working).

After leaving the U.S. Army Boxing Team in October 1986, I went to San Diego, California, to study sports massage therapy. My first chance to mix my newly learned sports massage therapy skills with my prior knowledge (much of which came from constant study, practice and learning from the Boxing Team doctor, Charles Pitluck D.O.), came when I teamed up with Dr. Keith Jeffers, a chiropractor that specialized in running injuries. While working there I learned a lot about the potential for soft tissue treatment, manipulation and exercise as a combination treatment approach.

About eighteen months later, I was the first massage therapist ever to be hired full time by a physical therapy clinic. I spent the next four years at "Sports and Orthopedic Physical Therapy" learning from and sharing my treatment philosophy with physical therapists, athletic trainers and orthopedic surgeons. During the five and a half years after I had left the Army, I spent a majority of my income on books and seminars. I traveled everywhere and anywhere to learn from the best osteopaths, physical therapists, chiropractors, medical doctors, athletic trainers, and movement and massage therapists. During this time, I had become quite successful at treating a host of chronic injuries in athletes and workers alike. I had also become well versed in kinesiology, biomechanics and modern injury care, as well as having developed a refined understanding of posture.

My next step in the developmental process was to open my own physical therapy clinic. Now, being licensed as a Holistic Health Practitioner made it impossible to practice P.T. and bill insurance companies, so I partnered with Steve Clark, P.T., M.S.S., M.B.A. Steve was a specialist in the knee, ankle and shoulder, which worked very well, as my specialty had grown to be spinal injuries, chronic injuries, head, neck and jaw pain, and sports conditioning. Over the next three and a half years, we ran our practice as the machine era continued to be in full swing...booming in fact!

It was routine practice for an athlete to ask, "Why didn't anyone ever teach us to lift weights this way?" when I was rehabilitating one of them at our clinic. The only answer I could provide was, "Money from machine sales and a body-building mentality are driving the industry, not the science of biomechanics or kinesiology!" As my success stories began to get around the industry, I was offered more and more consulting jobs with physical therapy clinics, professional sports teams and large companies. I was on a quest: *discover the truth about how the body works, how it should be cared for and get this information out to the people.*

In 1995, I began to see patients purely on a consulting basis so I could put my efforts into teaching seminars worldwide and making videotapes. By 1996, I had produced videos on core conditioning, back conditioning, and medicine ball training, and I had developed the first Swiss Ball training videos in the U.S. specifically for improving athletic performance. It wasn't until 1997 that I began to see light at the end of the tunnel—the exercise and rehabilitation industries were moving away from isokinetics and isolation machines, and into functional exercise. With this new light, came a new problem.

Functional exercise gurus began popping up like mushrooms in a cow pasture and many of them were taking the concept of functional exercise dangerously far! It was, and continues to be, a frank case of what Europeans would accuse someone of as "Americanism": if a little is good, then a lot must be better!

We now had experts traveling around the world demonstrating loaded lunges with rounded backs, claiming that to be functional, "the exercise must resemble the movement as closely as possible." For example, if you are a tennis player, you should lunge like you would reach for the ball, but do it under load. Although this approach has some "blind logic" to it, it is disrespectful of the fact that loading the musculoskeletal system in end range positions and postures is not something you want to do repetitiously unless you enjoy buying new cars for doctors! In a sporting event, your body will rarely ever be in exactly the same position under heavy load two times in a row. In the gym, performing the sports movement under load, over and over again, is insulting to joint mechanics and a great formula for injury!

Many of the same experts were ignorant of how to properly progress patients. In fact, I clearly remember seeing a presentation at the 1999 NSCA convention where one of the "functional exercise gurus" showed video footage of an athlete he was training to come back from an ACL injury; the athlete was doing various functional drills in sand, and to the trained eye, clearly demonstrated significant instability. This sort of thing has now become almost common place.

To keep functional exercise moving to the forefront of how we exercise and rehabilitate people, we must realize and follow a few key principles: All persons must be progressed forward in an exercise or rehabilitation program following the "flexibility/muscle balance—stability—strength—power" formula. This formula simply states that the first phase of an exercise or treatment program should focus on restoring optimal flexibility and muscle balance. The next phase is to train and condition the relevant stabilizers of the body. Next, building on the foundation of a now balanced and stable body, strength training can begin. Finally, after the body is balanced, stable and strong, power or high-speed training, can be implemented with minimal chance of iatrogenic (doctor/therapist/trainer induced) injury.

Movement speeds should progress from slow to moderate to fast. Intensities and load should always progress from lower to higher. If you isolate, you must integrate! This guideline simply suggests that in cases where isolation or bodybuilding type exercises are used (with the exception of bodybuilding for show only), the muscle developed must be integrated into functional movement via the use of functional exercises that incorporate that particular muscle. The movement pattern chosen for the purpose of integration should resemble both the pattern of injury and have a high level of carryover to the work or sport at hand for optimal integrative results.

Exercise order should always progress from the most to the least complex exercises. The only exception to the rule is when training elite athletes who are under the supervision of a trained professional. It is imperative to remember that the nervous system takes much longer to recover from an exercise than the musculature itself. Therefore, to get optimal performance and prevent unwanted injury, perform those exercises requiring the most cognitive and/or neural energy first.

Train, don't drain! When using functional exercises, we are generally performing exercises that require maintenance of one's center of gravity over one's own base of support. These exercises are much more taxing on the body and require much more mental energy and coordination. Performing these exercises with a bodybuilding mentality or "no pain, no gain" mentality only leads to "lots of pain and no gain!" Functional exercise is nervous system development exercise, or what I call software programming; if you put junk in the computer, that's exactly what will come out!

After over 16 years in orthopedic rehabilitation and sports conditioning, I can assure you that if we just follow these simple guidelines as we move into the functional exercise era, we will have less injury and our athletes will have a better chance of competing with athletes from countries that can't afford bodybuilding equipment!

—Paul Chek

— PREFACE —
THE WISDOM OF THE BODY
by Vern Gambetta

In today's high-tech world we sometimes forget the basics. The further away we go from the body, the less functional we become. The human body is a beautiful, finely tuned machine that far surpasses the most finely-tuned, high-performance technology known to man. It is the ultimate high-tech machine.

Despite all its complexity however, the body is also incredibly simple. Movement is a beautiful flow. The body has an inherent wisdom. In order to take advantage of the body's wisdom we must focus on how it functions. A thorough understanding of function will allow us to design and implement a very specific training program for each athlete we train. In order to understand function, we must understand movement.

The body is a link system; sometimes this link system is referred to as the kinetic chain. Functional training is all about linkage—it is about how all the parts of the chain work together in harmony to produce smooth, efficient patterns of movement. Most conventional academic preparation in Exercise and Movement Science focuses on studying individual muscles based on classical anatomy. This is where the confusion begins as to what is functional movement.

First of all, we must remember that we do not function in the anatomical position. The anatomical position is static and provides us only with an understanding of the arrangement of all the individual muscles. In many respects, learning about individual muscles is easier than learning about movement. *In order to truly understand function we must shift our focus from muscles to movements.* The brain does not recognize individual muscles. It recognizes patterns of movement, which consist of the individual muscles working in harmony to produce movement.

In order to further understand function we must understand the role that gravity plays. Gravity has minimal effect on the body in the anatomical position, but maximum effect on a body in motion. We simply cannot ignore gravity, it is essential for movement. It helps us to load the system. Therefore we must learn to overcome its effects, and to cheat and even defeat it occasionally. The fact that we live, work and play in a gravitationally enriched environment cannot be denied. Over reliance on machines gives us a false sense of security because they negate some of the effects of gravity. Gravity and its effects must be a prime consideration when designing and implementing a functional training program or we are not preparing the body for the forces that it must overcome.

How did I arrive at the point where the focus of my work is designing and implementing functional training programs for athletes in all sports? The key is my background as a track and field coach and my competitive background as a decathlete. The demands of track and field in terms of running, jumping and throwing encompass the whole spectrum of human movement. To be effective as a track coach, I learned early on that I had to train movements to get results. When I focused on isolated muscle actions I did not get the expected results—in fact I saw regression either in the form of performance decrement or injury.

For example, early in my coaching career I decided that I needed to strengthen the hamstrings more in order to help with sprinting speed. So I carefully designed a program that focused on isolating the hamstring through exercises that flexed the knee, such as the hamstring curl. Needless to say, the results were disastrous: several pulled hamstrings as well as persistent excessive tightness. Out of frustration I decided that I needed to find a better way. I realized that I needed to start by understanding what the hamstring really did in gait (when you're walking or running), not what the anatomy book told me. I found that in gait the hamstring works at the knee to decelerate the lower leg; at ground contact it works at the hip to extend the hip. Its minor function is to flex or bend the knee; in fact gravity and ground reaction forces play a much greater role in flexing the knee than does the hamstring. It is important to remember that the hamstring is a two-joint muscle, it works at both the knee and the hip. The way I was training the hamstring, I was training it as a one joint muscle, isolating the hamstring as a flexor of the knee. This created neural confusion. In essence I was sending a mixed message to the hamstring. I was telling it to do one thing in training and then asking it to do something entirely different when we were sprinting. This is typical of programs that follow conventional wisdom.

The lesson that I learned from this was to always carefully look at the movement that I was trying to enhance and to ask the following questions: What are the forces involved? What is the dominant plane of motion? How does that muscle fit in as a link in the whole kinetic chain? For example, at the hamstring the emphasis switched to lunges and step-ups, which work the hamstring muscle group in a functional manner. *It is imperative to understand the movements and then design the training program accordingly.*

Another major pitfall that I had to learn to avoid was the trap of emphasizing measurable strength. How much you can lift or how many foot-pounds of force you can express on a dynamometer are meaningless numbers. The key is how you use that strength. How is the force expressed? Can you produce and reduce the force? Force production is all about acceleration, but often the key to movement efficiency and staying injury free is the ability to decelerate—which is the ability to reduce force. A good functional training program will work on the interplay between force production and force reduction. The end result is functional strength.

Ultimately, the glue that binds a whole functional program together is proprioception. Proprioception is awareness of joint position derived from feedback in the sense receptors in the joints, ligaments, tendons, and muscles. It is a highly trainable quality that we have tended to take for granted. It is almost too simple. Perhaps to appreciate proprioception we should look at the extreme case of a stroke victim that is able to return to normal movement patterns. Why can't athletes who have all their capacities enhance the quality of their movement by focusing on the same things that the stroke victim has to focus on to get back to function? The key to that is proprioception. We must strive to constantly change proprioceptive demand throughout the training program.

Understanding and training functionally is a challenging process. It is often contrary to conventional wisdom as represented in current mainstream sport science research. In order to move forward this should not limit us. We need to use conventional wisdom as a starting point and move forward faster, higher and stronger. Good luck following the functional path, I hope it is as much fun for you as it has been for me.

—Vern Gambetta

— INTRODUCTION —
A REVOLUTIONARY APPROACH TO FITNESS
by RoseMarie Alfieri

Fitness for fitness sake is out. Gone are the days of going to the gym just to buff up and look good. Today, many people want to get fit for a specific reason other than aesthetics: they want to accomplish specific goals such as hike a mountain, improve their golf game or to perform specific daily tasks with greater ease. Take the following cases for example:

Martha, a New York City businesswoman in her fifties, loves ballroom dancing and wanted to improve her stamina and technique.

Lisa, a thirty-two-year-old competitive cyclist was anxious to begin cycle cross racing, a challenging closed-loop bike race that involves overcoming obstacles.

And, Roger—a fifty-seven-year-old former dancer—wanted to learn how to turn his dancing acumen into a quick one-two punch in the boxing ring.

Martha, Lisa and Roger differ in age, occupation and interests, but have at least one thing in common: each has incorporated functional training into his or her fitness program in order to meet specific goals and objectives. And they have done so with great success. "I wish I knew about functional training when I was an athlete in school," says Lisa. "All we did then was run, practice and lift weights. I am so much more fit now!"

The term functional training has become somewhat of a buzzword in the last couple of years and has popped up in health clubs across the country where boot camp classes, plyometric work, sports circuits, and balance and stability training abound. It is important to note that while it has recently become a buzzword, and as such risks being categorized as merely the trend of the moment, biomechanical research and the fitness experts interviewed for this book agree that in fact it represents *a true revolution in the ways in which we work out.* The American Council on Exercise, a national non-profit fitness certification and education organization, predicts that the next decade will see a major increase in training that is functionally oriented. That's because functional training allows your body to work the way it was meant to; it truly conditions your body to be stronger and fit, and is specific to whatever your exercise goal may be. It is also especially relevant to older adults who, after years of being sedentary or of doing traditional exercise in the gym that is not functional, find that the physical activities of daily life: climbing stairs, getting in and out of the car, carrying groceries, etc. have become increasingly challenging.

Whether you are new to working out or have been a gym rat for years, functional training is an important type of training that should be incorporated into your workout program. It is the training of today and of tomorrow. *So what exactly is this revolutionary form of exercise?*

There are several ways to define functional training. For now a brief definition is provided, with more in-depth discussion to follow in Chapter One. Simply put, functional training requires you to move your body as a complete integrated unit, working many muscles at the same time—just as you would in daily life. Think about it. When you walk to work, run to catch a train or bus, or lift a box or bag of groceries, you are not just using one muscle. You are using many that work in concert to execute the desired action. Vern Gambetta, former coach of the Chicago White Sox, and one of the experts interviewed for this book, reminds us to "keep in mind that the body works as a kinetic chain, with force both produced and reduced during movement." This is the opposite of traditional bodybuilding where you concentrate on isolating a body part (for example, doing a preacher curl for the biceps or using the leg extension machine for your quadriceps). Because it requires balance, stability and the use of your core muscles—in particular your abdominals, pelvis girdle and lower back—functional training is exceptionally efficient. It works a lot in a short amount of time. And, not only does it make you stronger, it makes your body more flexible and stable too. It can help you meet your fitness goals faster and better than other types of training.

While this may all sound good, you may be wondering if it is really necessary. After all, you may already be working out at the gym a few times a week, lifting or benching a challenging weight. Or you may run regularly and feel that you're in good condition. Your body fat levels might be low and your cardiovascular capacity strong. Why change your routine? Well, in addition to the fact that cross training is important to stimulate your muscles differently and to avoid hitting a workout plateau, functional training is considered by many, including the experts in this book, essential to prevent injury and to attain "fitness" that goes beyond being skin deep. It gets to the "core" of things. Both CC Cunningham, owner of PerformEnhance and a member of the Life Fitness Academy, and Paul Chek, founder of the C.H.E.K. Institute, use automobile analogies to describe the differences between having a souped-up exterior (big muscles) and having a really strong, well running engine (a powerful core).

Functional training—while not neglecting muscles and muscle development—focuses heavily on developing and maintaining a powerful core.

In addition, Chek has noted a tidal shift in the general public's perception of the effectiveness of the non-functional workouts that they have been doing for years—especially in the baby boomer population. "People are getting wise to what works and what doesn't work," Chek says, and are "coming to the harsh conclusion that a lot of the equipment is garbage." While these people are saying that they look great, they are biomechanical wrecks, with aches and pains galore. An individualized functional training program can correct the imbalances caused by years of isolation training.

Convinced?

Well, perhaps knowing the following will do it for you. Nearly everyone who regularly exercises at some point or another grows bored with his or her exercise programs. They become, alas, routine. Instead of looking forward to your morning jog or weight lifting circuit, you fret about how long the session will take and what you'll be doing afterwards. Taking a functional training approach to fitness will help alleviate that boredom. Why? Because, FUNctional training has a very high FUN component:

> **It Frees you** from the repetitious nature of isolation machine-based exercises, offering a great deal of variety in terms of both the types of exercise you can do and the equipment you can use; and because it involves the simultaneous recruitment of multiple muscles, it is time-efficient.

> **It is Useful,** helping your body to get stronger and more fit not only so you can look great as you flex your muscles in the gym (although, of course that may be one of your fitness goals), but so you can perform every day activities as well as the sports and leisure time activities that you enjoy and look forward to with greater ease and success.

> **It is Necessary.** Without using our muscles and brains in an integrated, synergistic way eventually we will lose stability, performance capability, fitness and ultimately, the independence to take care of ourselves. If you are not training in a functional manner, you are at risk for these problems, regardless of how good you look or how good you currently feel.

And so, in short, functional training is something everyone must do to preserve independence and achieve true fitness.

While you may now be intrigued, undoubtedly you have several questions about functional training and how to develop a program that is right for you.

Like all self improvement processes in life, your functional training program is a journey, with this book providing your first step along the road to total whole body fitness. It is for everyone of all ages and fitness levels.

Specifically, this book includes the following:

In-depth information on functional training, the equipment you can use, and how to differentiate it from other types of exercise to help you to determine what is and what is not considered functional.

Research and expert opinions about the benefits of functional training and the general principles of functional training programs so you can custom tailor a program to fit your needs.

Several goal-specific subcategories. Each subcategory features a renowned fitness expert, who provides his or her philosophy of functional training as well as a specially designed program just for you. The experts and their subcategories are:

Michael Jenniex, MA, is program director for the Whitaker Wellness Center in Naples, Fla., and a fitness educator for Exercise Etc. He currently is the strength coach for Florida Gulf Coast University and the pro trainer for the Southeast region for Bodytraining Systems. Mike provides his views in Chapter Three on flexibility training's role in functional fitness.

Paul Chek, MMS, NMT, HHP, is a top expert in the area of functional fitness and is an internationally acclaimed speaker and consultant in the fitness field. He has authored several books, videos and correspondence courses and is founder of the C.H.E.K. Institute in San Diego, Calif., which provides education and certification for exercise professionals worldwide. Chek kicks off the functional training programs with a core training program in Chapter Four.

Annette Lang, MA, develops and teaches personal trainer education programs throughout the country for the Esquerre Fitness Group and Reebok University. In Chapter Five she provides a program to help prepare you for activities for daily life.

Christine (CC) Cunningham, MS, specializes in athlete development. She is the owner of PerformEnhance sports performance training in Evanston, Ill., and is a member of the Life Fitness Academy. CC, a doctoral candidate in Exercise Neuroscience at the University of Illinois, presents a functional strength-training program in Chapter Six.

Vern Gambetta, MA, is the director of Gambetta Training Systems. Gambetta is renowned in the field of athletic training, having served as the speed and conditioning coach for the Tampa Bay Mutiny Major League Soccer Team from 1996–1999 and as conditioning consultant to the U.S. Men's World Cup Team and New England Revolution in 1998. In addition, he is the former Director of Conditioning for the Chicago White Sox. Recognized the world over as an expert in training and conditioning for sports, he has worked with world-class athletes and teams in a wide variety of sports. In Chapter Seven he provides you with a program to improve athletic performance.

Paul Frediani, ACSM, is a nationally recognized fitness trainer and educator, certified by the American College of Sports Medicine and the American Council on Exercise. A former Golden Gloves Champion who is affiliated with Equinox Health Club in New York, and president of BoxAthletics, Frediani shows you in Chapter Eight how to use a great tool—the medicine ball—to get the most from your functional workouts.

Finally, the book provides guidelines to help you develop a manageable, personal, goal-based workout program that incorporates functional training.

Ready?

Good. Sit back, start reading and begin your first step, or jog, or run along the road to functional training and a happier, healthier lifestyle.

CHAPTER 1

WHAT IS FUNCTIONAL TRAINING?

WHICH IS FUNCTIONAL?

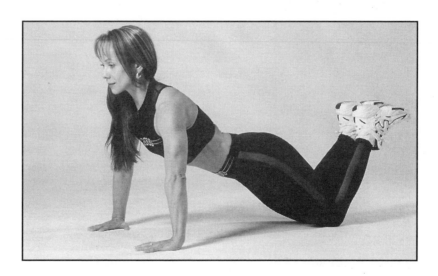

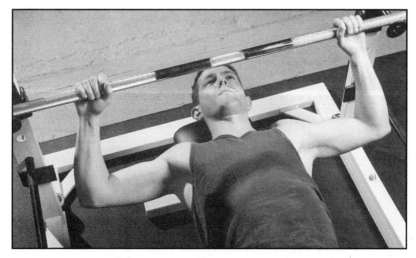

A push-up versus a bench press?

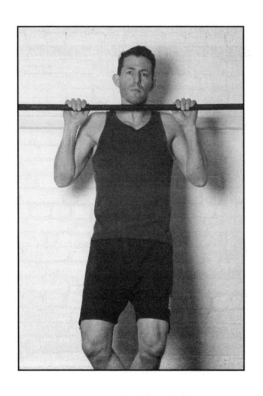 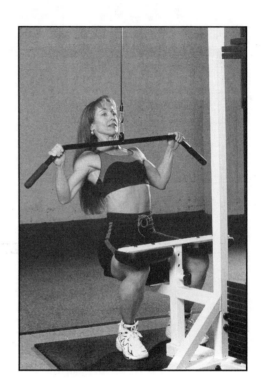

A pull-up versus the lat pull down machine?

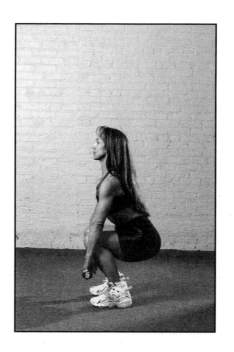

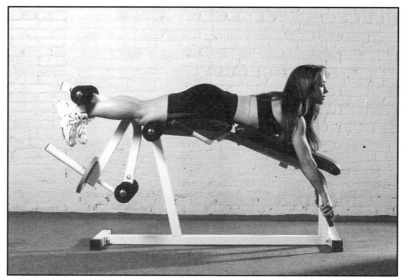

A squat versus a hamstring curl machine?

FUNCTIONAL TRAINING

The exercises on the previous pages present functional exercises as well as those typically not categorized as functional. Do you know which are which? If you selected the pull-up, push-up and squat as the more functional exercises, you are correct. Why? Because the pull-up, push-up and squat all move the body in multiple planes and as an integrated unit. They integrate rather than isolate your muscles. They don't rely on the assistance that machines provide. Functional training is differentiated from other types of programs, such as bodybuilding. The goal of functional training *is to increase body awareness and overall strength and conditioning, so that we can transfer these gains to better performance of daily life activities and/or sports.*

THE BASICS OF FUNCTIONAL TRAINING

According to The American Council on Exercise (ACE), "Functional training requires an integration of balance and intrinsic muscular stability during the exertion of muscular force and often uses closed chain movement."[1] Closed chain movement will be explained a bit later in this chapter. In addition to ACE's definition, several of the fitness experts who present their programs in this book have their own conceptions about functional training.

Vern Gambetta provides a concise definition that we can analyze to truly understand the concepts behind functional training. According to Gambetta, "Functional exercise is integrated, multi-dimensional movement that requires acceleration, deceleration and stabilization in all three planes." Let's take this definition apart to understand fully what it means.

Use Integrated Movement

Integrated movement means that we do not train by isolating muscles. For example when we work the biceps using a biceps curl machine, we are supporting our entire body by resting against the machine, and not allowing our own body's stabilizing muscles in the back, stomach and legs to work to stabilize us. Therefore, we are isolating all the work in the biceps. In functional training, we work the body in such a way that it recruits several muscles (as in a pull-up, which hits the lats, biceps, abdominals, lower back and shoulders). Each muscle performs a different function (accelerating, decelerating, or stabilizing) in order to successfully achieve the desired movement.

This concept is very different from traditional bodybuilding, which is the sport for which gyms were built, and around which an entire industry—including several magazines, movies and books—bloomed (think Arnold). Bodybuilders isolate muscles and use heavy resistance in order to obtain a great deal of hypertrophy, which is a fancy word for enlarged muscle. As a sport, bodybuilding is not concerned with developing a body that as an entire unit can function to its maximum capacity; instead it is more concerned with developing individual muscular strength and with aesthetics: how ripped or toned the body appears.

In contrast, when we do functional training we don't take our bodies apart muscle by muscle, we work our whole person. Indeed, the resounding message or theme at the ECA World Fitness Conference, held in New York, April 2000, *was integrate: don't isolate and work your core!*

Get off the Machines

Because we want to integrate not isolate, and because we want the movement to be multi-dimensional, the value of working out on machines is seriously questioned by many in the functional training field. In general, because machines offer so much external support—on many you are in a seated position with your back fully supported—they do not challenge your body in a functional way.

Think about the leg press machine. Your back is entirely supported, and your abdominals don't have to work hard to stabilize your body as they normally would because you are lying down–an unnatural position for movement in the real world. Compare this to doing a standing squat exercise with free weights or a single bar on your back. Not only are your quadriceps, gluteals (buttocks) and hamstrings working when you squat, you also must use your lower back muscles and abdominals to balance and stabilize your body so that you don't tip over. In their article "Training Principles," authors Michael and Margaret Stone, reviewed research done on machine and free weight training. They found that while it is possible to change weight intensity with machines, "proper application, sequencing and variation of movement patterns, speed-strength and speed-oriented exercises are limited at best. This is due to the limitations in the movement pattern and movement characteristics of the machines themselves."[2] In other words, *the machines will help you grow big muscles, but will not help you apply that growth in the real world—whether that be in a sport or in a daily life activity.*

That is why using free weights for training is considered more functional than using machines, and explains why you generally can lift a lot heavier resistance with machines than you can with dumbbells. Annette Lang puts it this way: "Free weights are harder because the body must stabilize. Think about how much weight you could lift on a one-arm seated row machine—totally supported—as compared to a classic single arm row with your knee bent on a bench; and then compare that to a single arm row with total self stabilization." The last version of this exercise for your back is the most challenging and because you must use your stabilizing muscles to balance when you do the row, you will not be able to lift as much weight as you can with the machine or with the partial support of a bench. *So while you might be lifting lighter weight, you're actually working harder.*

While many experts in the functional training field believe that you should start off right away with free weights, some experts, such as CC Cunningham, feel that there is a place for machine training in functional training: namely to correct a muscular imbalance. For example, if you have a weak left bicep, you may want to use an isolation exercise to make it stronger before you do traditional functional exercise. You also may use the assistance of machines to build up to self-stabilization if you are just beginning to learn a movement and need to focus on one thing at a time, before it becomes automatic. And, of course if your goal is bodybuilding, then isolation training is for you. But that's another book.

Move in Multi-Planes

We can move our bodies in three directional ways or planes: we can bend side to side, which is called moving in the lateral or frontal plane; we can bend forward or backward, which is moving in the saggital plane; and we can twist at the waist, which is moving in the transverse plane. Why is moving in several planes functional? Most of the activities that we have to do every day, such as bending down to pick up an object, or reaching at an angle to retrieve a can from a high cupboard, require us to move in a combination of planes. And, all athletic sports require that your body be agile in its movements in many planes. Think of a golfer who uses twisting actions as well as flexes and extends several muscles during a swing.

To further understand functional training, consider acclaimed expert Paul Chek's philosophy. Chek, who presents a core training program in Chapter Four, focuses on strengthening and conditioning the body's core muscles: the abdominals, spine, pelvis and diaphragm. He also presents some great stability exercises that are both static (not moving) and dynamic (when moving).

Condition Your Core

What works harder in the course of a day, your core (midsection) or your arms and legs? Most of us probably would guess the arms and legs. After all, we are constantly swinging our arms, moving our hands and using our legs. In fact, in terms of functionality, the arms and legs are like amateur body builders, and the core an Olympic power lifter—because it has to do so much at all times.

The body's core serves so many functions. As Chek explains, it protects our internal organs, protects our nervous system and spinal cord, and serves as the "body's primary pump" to circulate blood from the heart to the extremities as well as the body's system for stabilization and movement. The body's core provides the attachment points for our extremities, the arms and legs. Chek calls the core the "key region" of our bodies, which acts as a "force conductor." Essentially, all of the movement that our bodies generate does not come from the legs, but from the action of the core muscles, which provide an integrated stabilizing action that allows movement to be transferred to and from our legs. In addition, the spine is involved. According to Chek, rather than being a passive column as often it is thought of, the spine in fact acts as an engine that helps to propel your legs and arms into action. Unfortunately, most traditional gym exercises do nothing to condition this vital part of our bodies—the part that is the genesis of all of our function. And, our sedentary society has produced a nation of people who are both soft and stagnant around the middle from sitting so much of the day. As Annette Lang puts it, all the conveniences of the technological age has "bred a society that doesn't need the stability of the core." *So, true functional training entails working the entire core area, both inner and outer, to achieve a stable, strong and powerful force to safely perform all movement.*

Do Closed Chain Exercises

Annette Lang considers exercises functional "when you are moving your own body through space." Here is where the difference between a closed chain and an open chain exercise becomes apparent. As the ACE definition states, functional training often uses closed chain movement. Closed chain exercises are those that closely resemble human movement, in which the end of the chain of movement is fixed against the floor and supports the weight of the body (for example doing a squat or lunge). The way your muscles are recruited and the joint movements of closed chain exercises differ greatly from open chain exercises, with closed chain movements crucial to improving performance.[3] In an open chain exercise the fixed point is at your hip (usually you are seated in a machine) and the end of the chain is open or free (for example a leg extension machine where you are strapped into an upright seat and bend and extend your leg out into space). Closed chain exercises work more muscles, help your body perform better during daily activities and increase neuromuscular awareness of your body.

Transfer Your Training

CC Cunningham likes to think of functional training in terms of "transfer training" meaning that the exercises you do in the gym or at home can directly help you to be better at daily life activities, such as gardening or lifting groceries, or can help your performance in a sport or athletic activity you enjoy—whether it be your golf game, tennis, or hiking. To achieve this kind of transfer effect, the brain has to come into play, which can be a bit complicated to understand. Simply put, all of our muscles have receptors that transmit signals to the brain, which in turn trigger the brain to execute a "move" command. The brain must recognize the movement done during the exercise as being exactly the same as the movement that you want to perform better in daily life or in a sport.

Why? Because of the law of specificity, *which states that in order to get better at a physical activity—whether it be running, playing tennis or golf—the exercise must be as similar as possible to the actual activity in several ways.* These ways include coordination, range of motion, type of contraction and speed of movement.[4] In other words, not only should the type of resistance used in the exercise be identical to the resistance used in the actual activity, so should the movement patterns, peak force and the velocity, or speed with which you perform the exercise. In traditional strength training programs little transfer occurs. Think about it. If you are in the gym and try to mimic a golf swing with a dumbbell, you are not helping your game because the weight is not exactly the same as the club and you handle it differently. So, if your goal is to swing a 10 or 20 pound weight around great, but if it's to improve your golf game? Sorry, won't happen. More on the important issue of transfer appears in the next chapter.

So now you know the basics of what makes an exercise functional: using integrated rather than isolated movement of muscles, moving in more than one plane, recruiting and conditioning the core muscles, performing more closed chain than open chain exercises and doing exercises so that they produce a transfer effect.

TYPES OF FUNCTIONAL TRAINING

Because functional training is concerned with exercise that will mean something to you outside of the gym, we have broken it down into several subcategories, each of which are related to a specific goal. Decide which areas are weak spots for you and then read the corresponding chapter to learn how to turn a weakness into strength.

Flexibility

Poor flexibility. It so often is the neglected stepsister when it comes to our exercise programs. But its importance should never be underestimated. A flexible body is like a well-oiled machine and will take you far in your quest to be strong, fit and resistant to injury.

Core Conditioning and Stability

Where would we be without our cores? Essentially, we'd just be a head with a bunch of flailing limbs. If you've been doing your standard crunches and reverse curls for years and think your center is as strong as can be, think again AND review the chapter on core conditioning. You'll soon be moving in new, more effective ways toward real core strength.

Activities for Daily Life

Just being alive requires us to move—even during these very sedentary technologically driven times. We still need to walk, and on occasion run or sprint: most of us have, at one time or another, missed a bus or train and had to make a dash for it, with briefcase and donut in hand. Functional training can be geared toward improving the functions needed to remain independent: such as the ability to push and pull and to lift and lower. Anyone at any age who wants to be able to move through life a little easier, sans aches and pains, should perform exercises to help with activities for daily life.

Functional Strength Training

Strength training that achieves a transfer effect is functional and looks very different from the traditional weight lifting training that you have probably seen at the gym. If you want to gain strength in ways that ensure you can take what you learn out of the gym and into the garden or onto the court, you need to do functional strength training.

Programs for Athletic Performance

Want to score more goals, swing a longer drive or beat your best time in the 5K run? Then you want to pursue functional training programs that are sports-specific and which involve training for power, agility and coordination. These programs, through analysis of movement patterns and simulation, can help you be better at whatever your favorite game is.

TOOLS OF THE TRADE

Because functional training involves moving and using your body in very real-life, multi-directional ways, you can get an effective workout without using any equipment. The resistance of your own body weight will help you to attain gains in strength through exercises such as push ups, pull-ups and squats.

That said, there are a variety of tools and products—many of which are essential components of a physical therapist's "tool box"—that you can incorporate in your training program to specifically challenge your body to work functionally, and which target balance, coordination, and agility, in particular. Plus, the variety makes training fun and different each time you work out.

Here's a rundown of some of the most popular functional training products, some of which are used by our experts in the workouts they have designed for you. See the appendix for information on where you can obtain these and other fantastic training tools.

> *Unstable Surfaces:* These include beams, wobble and rocker boards, foam rollers, and pads, which provide unstable surfaces that force your body to stabilize and align properly, and help you to use your body as a complete unit.

> *Balls:* Medicine Ball, Stability Ball, Resist-A-Ball. The medicine ball, which comes in a variety of weights helps you to apply strength to athletic performance. Stability Balls and Resist-A-Balls, which come in various sizes depending upon your height,

have unstable contours that improve your body alignment, stability, strength and flexibility, and are ideal for core training.

Ladder & Rings: The ABC ladder is a staple for agility and coordination training. This nylon ladder is placed on the floor; the challenge is to hop, run, walk, etc. between the rungs to improve speed and agility and to increase proprioceptive awareness. Multicolored fitness rings that look a bit like the fitness fad Hula Hoop of years gone by, can be used for a number of drills to develop speed, balance, reaction and endurance.

Tubing/Bands: There are a number of different tubing and band products available that add external resistance to your workouts while helping you to train your body to stabilize and balance.

Free Weights: Of course, free weights provide functional weight training because your body has to stabilize itself and balance on many planes when you are doing a standing exercise with dumbbells.

Now you've got a basic understanding of the concepts and types of functional training, but before we delve into our experts' training programs, let's first turn our attention to relevant research on this topic, the general principles or guidelines for functional training programs and specific benefits you can get from this type of workout.

There is a wide variety of equipment you can use for functional training to keep it fun, diverse and interesting. The equipment helps you to achieve such functional goals as training your core muscles, improving strength, coordination and athletic performance, and improving your body's ability to balance.

1. Stability ball
2. Medicine ball
3. Balance board
4. Free weights
5. Jump rope
6. Step

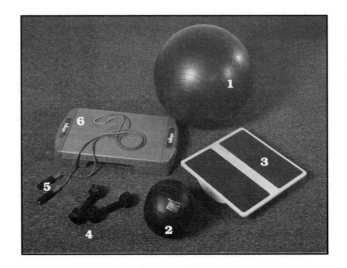

CHAPTER 2

PRINCIPLES OF FUNCTIONAL TRAINING

A FITNESS BOOM

Functional training is hot hot hot! Look around everywhere and you'll see "tools of the trade"—stability balls, ladders and tubing literally cluttering up gyms throughout the country. And you thought your home was a mess! While this type of training certainly is revolutionary and represents a paradigm shift in how people like you perceive fitness, there's really nothing new about it. In fact, it is a perfect example of the expression "everything old is new again."

The roots of functional training are in physical therapy and rehabilitation. For decades physical therapists have used medicine balls, stability balls and balance boards with their clients, helping to restore their bodies to a level of function that was lost due to an accident, injury, genetic problem, aging or some other traumatic event. Then in the past few years, functional training began to travel "mainstream" to the gyms and health clubs from two distinct sources.

First, personal trainers increasingly were approached by clients who were coming off an injury, had finished their physical therapy, and wanted to get back into shape. Many of these clients were baby boomers who had spent year after year doing high impact exercises such as running and aerobics, or who had gotten involved in heavy weight lifting and were suffering the cumulative effects of repetitive stress and imbalance. In fact, often the clients would come to the trainers with specific exercises prescribed by their physical therapists. The old lifting model of training (bodybuilding) would not work for these clients and consequently, trainers began to investigate and incorporate functional exercises with these clients. Once trainers and clients saw the great results of such training, they began to incorporate aspects of it in general with all of their clients.

The second way that functional training got into health clubs was in the area of sports conditioning. Vern Gambetta believes that the high levels of performance that athletes have is the model that people look at ultimately. They begin to ask: What does that baseball player, marathon runner or golfer do that enables him or her to be so good at a sport? And, they want to do that, too. For years coaches have used functional training, without labeling it as such in the form of agility and coordination drills, power work and dynamic stability training—all techniques that use the whole body rather than isolate muscles.

But traditionally the fitness industry in general did not focus on this type of training. Says Annette Lang, "We in the fitness industry thought we didn't need to take people from the aerobic room into agility training. We used to think 'they don't need this because they are not athletes'." Well times have changed. Lang notes that now many people want to get fit for a specific purpose that goes beyond looking good in a bathing suit. They want to relate their fitness to the demands of the sport or activity they enjoy.

PRINCIPLES OF FUNCTIONAL TRAINING PROGRAMS

There is most definitely a science to functional training. While you may be anxious to jump in and embrace a functional training program without getting into all the technical mumbo jumbo, it is important for you to have a basic comprehension of the biomechanics (how the structures or parts of our bodies move according to the physical laws of motion) of functional training. With this understanding, you will be able to determine for yourself whether an exercise you are doing is functional as well as how to design your own functional training program.

Recognize the Brain Connection

First, know that every single task that we do, whether it be walking, dancing or even smiling actually involves the performance of many skills and gets down to the cellular level. Neurons are cells that receive and send messages through our central nervous system to our brain. There are certain neurons, called motor neurons that innervate your muscle fibers. Each motor neuron and the muscle fibers it stimulates form what is known as a motor unit. Motor units are responsible for exerting force and hence making a part of your body (be it a leg or arm) move. Messages from neurons transmitted through the central nervous system tell our brain what type of movement to execute. So, in effect all exercise is really quite a "brainy" endeavor as no movement is possible without a good working relationship between the central nervous system and our muscles.[1]

In functional training we are concerned with another concept known as proprioception, which is defined as the perception of the positions of our body parts. Essentially, this means your awareness of your body in terms of posture, movement, equilibrium and position. As Paul Chek writes in *The Golf Biomechanics Manual*, it is the brain's ability to sense movement.[2] These sensations are perceived through receptors in your joints, tendons and muscles. If you have good proprioception, the signals moving from the brain to the muscles are sharp and focused, and you will have good control of your body. As CC Cunningham puts it, "You have to understand what the brain uses as signals to the muscles." The role of your neurological system is vital to achieve what we briefly discussed in Chapter One, namely "Transfer of Training" to a real life activity.

How to Transfer Your Training

While this book provides some sample workouts to develop functional fitness, the very nature of functional fitness is individualized. The goals of a competitive athlete are most likely very different from those of someone who wants to improve his or her weekend sport or who wants to be better at lifting objects in every day life. Therefore the exercises that you will do will depend upon your own personal goals and abilities, and your base fitness level. Because of this individuality, it will be very helpful for you to learn how to determine whether an exercise is functional for you. This way, you can maximize the efficiency of your workouts and will be able to design your own customized training program. *In other words, you won't waste time on exercises that aren't related to your goals and objectives!*

If you want your workouts to help you be better at something else—whether to perform daily tasks or to improve your mountain biking skills—what you're really saying is that you want your gym or home workout to TRANSFER to that other activity. There are certain things that your workout must contain in order for this to happen. *Most important is that the exercise must be as similar as possible to the actual activity.* This makes sense and holds true not only for functional training, but really for anything you want to do. For example, if you want to be a better piano player, you need to play a keyboard instrument—ideally, a piano. You know, practice makes perfect! You certainly wouldn't become a better piano player by learning the flute, although it may help you develop your overall sense of musicality. Similarly, if you want to be a better biker and think that your 60 minutes run on the treadmill is going to do it, you may be in for disappointment. Your run may improve your cardiovascular system and burn tons of calories, but to be a better biker you simply have to bike or strengthen your biking muscles (quadriceps, gluteals, hamstrings) by working them in ways that simulate biking. *The closer the exercise is to your actual physical performance, the greater the likelihood that you will transfer strength and fitness gains to that activity.*[3]

So, to try to make sure that the exercises you do mimic as closely as possible your desired activity, you need to concentrate on making them as similar as possible in the following four areas:

> **Coordination:** This is your ability to coordinate the timing of your muscle contractions, so that they are similar to contractions of your goal activity. Coordination also means that we are using integrated body movement rather than isolation, because you must train all the body parts that are involved in your goal movement. Cunningham offers the following example, "Suppose you want to improve your golf swing so you decide to use tubing to

mimic the movement pattern. However, if you think about it, in a real golf swing your muscles contract hardest in the upswing and then decelerate at the bottom. With tubing, you are doing the opposite-your muscles will contract hardest at the bottom of the swing. Therefore, an exercise you think will help improve your golf swing ends up messing up your movement pattern."

Range of Motion: Range of motion is the length of the movement from beginning to endpoint. So, for a golf swing, it would be the distance from the upswing to the downswing. If you are doing functional exercises that imitate your swing, you need to perform them with the same (or greater) range of motion as you would on the links. According to Cunningham, "In training, each joint involved in the movement should progress through the same range of motion as in the goal movement."

Type: You must use the same type of contraction as you would use in your goal movement. The major types of contractions include concentric contractions (when your muscles get shorter as you contract. Example: bending your arms at the elbow during a biceps curl), eccentric contractions (when your muscles get longer against the resistance. Example: lowering or extending your arms in a biceps curl), and isometric contractions (when there is no perceivable movement. Example: holding a squat position).

Speed: Finally, the speed at which you perform your exercises should be the same as the speed of your goal activity or movement.[4]

When trying to develop a functional exercise given your own particular goal, you also need to ask yourself the following questions:

1.   **What joints are involved in the movement and how do the muscles work** (what type of contraction-isometric (stabilizing), concentric, eccentric)?

2.   **What is the range of motion at each joint during the activity and the exercise?**

3.   **What is the speed of the contraction?**

4.   **What kind of equipment can I use to help me to copy the movement?**

Then, try to do an exercise that mimics each of these areas.

THE IMPORTANCE OF PROGRESSION

If there is one resounding message that our experts stress above all else, it is this: in order for your functional training program to be both effective and safe you must follow certain rules of progression. What does this mean? Well, just as you had to crawl before you walked and walked before you ran, you need to build your functional training in phases. Because functional training involves using many muscles and movement patterns at the same time, you need to learn the exercises in stages.

If you have never done a lunge before, the last thing you want to do is grab two eight-pound dumbbells and try to perform backward lunges off a raised platform. Your body and brain will be trying to do too many things at once: stabilizing your core muscles as you try to lunge back, contracting the gluteals and quadriceps, etc., all while trying not to fall off the bench! Way too much to process!

You've probably seen people at the gym—most often in a "one size fits all" body sculpting class where an instructor has 20 people all doing complicated movements like the lunge off a bench—whose form is terrible (they are leaning over or wobbling from side to side and look like any moment they will topple over). Simply, they should not be doing this particular exercise yet, because their neuromuscular system has not yet learned how to perform all these movements at the same time. First, they should focus on stability exercises and strengthening their core, then on coordination. Once they can perform the lunge in good form, with proper alignment and posture (not leaning forward or backward), then they can try to add weights. Since all of our bodies are differ-

---

HOW FAT ARE YOU?

The numbers on the scale may seem good, but did you know you can be a normal weight and yet overfat at the same time? To determine your body composition (the percentage of your body's mass that comes from fat) you need to have a skinfold caliper test performed on you by a fitness professional. Here are ACE's guidelines for body fat percentages in men and women.

Classification	Women	Men
Essential Fat	10-12%	2-4%
Athletes	14-20%	6-13%
Fitness	25-31%	18-25%
Acceptable	25-31%	18-25%
Obese	32 +	25+

Source: **Lifestyle & Weight Management Consultant Manual**, The American Council on Exercise (ACE), 1996.

ent—some of us are more flexible than others, have stronger cores or longer legs—we must each build progression, according to our individual needs. Here are some general rules:

- Begin without weights or extra resistance and gradually add resistance.
- Begin on a stable surface, such as a floor and progress to an unstable one, such as a wobble board.
- First work on stability and coordination.
- Perform the exercise slowly with a lot of control; you can speed it up once you've mastered it.

BENEFITS OF FUNCTIONAL TRAINING

There are so many benefits to functional training. Overall, they include gains in strength, power, coordination, agility and balance. These gains all are related to improving your ability to be physically active without injuring yourself— therefore improving your quality of life.

We close this chapter with some of the specific benefits of functional training:

Results Transfer to Real Life: The high degree of specificity involved in functional training leads to greater transfer of gains to your sport of choice or everyday activity. *You'll be better at what you want/love to do!*

More Calories Burned: Because functional training uses big muscle movements and does a lot at the same time, these exercises require more energy than isolation exercises. Therefore, they are more likely to elevate metabolism than traditional exercises, which leads to more lean body mass and less fat. *So, if your goal is to improve your body composition (that is the percentage of your body that is lean) functional training provides an effective, efficient approach to shaping a better body.*

Time Saved: In functional training, unlike with machine weight training, you move quickly from exercise to exercise and work out your whole body instead of working it out in segments. *This translates into results with less expenditure of time.*

Cost Lowered: When you do functional training, you don't need to use big (expensive) machines. Many of the exercises can be done with just your own body weight or with dumbbells and small, relatively inexpensive props like a stability ball or balance board. *You save money!*

CHAPTER 3

FLEXIBILITY TRAINING

Why is flexibility important for developing functional fitness? Flexibility is your body's ability to move within a range of motion. So much of what we do in daily life as well as in athletics is dependent on how flexible we are. "If you pick something up off the floor, you involve flexibility of your hamstring," explains Mike Jenniex, program director for Whitaker Wellness Center in Naples, Fla., international fitness educator, and strength coach for Florida Gulf Coast University. "Flexibility training is really one of the most functional things you can do for your workout program," Mike explains.

Most people know that fitness professionals, industry organizations and even doctors, recommend a stretching or flexibility program, but it seems always to be given the short end of the workout stick. We may spend over an hour running, biking or doing strength training and then *maybe*, just maybe, shove in five minutes of stretching at the end. Too often the stretching segment of our workouts is rushed and not as effective as it should and could be. We're bored with exercising by that point and just want to get on with whatever else we need to do. When we do this however, we cheat ourselves of the many benefits of flexibility training. They include: increased range of motion around a joint, decreased risk of injury, and better physical performance. Time spent stretching is time well spent. In fact, Mike recommends that flexibility training be done every day.

TYPES OF STRETCHING

There are several different types of stretching programs you can do. Most of you probably are familiar with static stretching-the long sustained stretch you hold after a workout. But this is just one form of flexibility training. In general, flexibility programs are classified as either passive or active. Static stretching is passive. Active programs include ballistic stretching, PNF stretching, active warm-ups, and active-isolated stretching. Active flexibility programs are directly related to the neurological and physiological function at hand. In other words, there is coordination between the opposing muscles at a joint that makes this type of stretch more in-depth than a passive stretch.

Mike recommends first getting a full analysis of your postural alignment by a fitness professional to determine where you may have flexibility problems. He also emphasizes that you must determine what benefit you want to get from the increased flexibility. For example, if you are a basketball player and want to improve your game performance you will want to make sure that your stretching program includes active stretches. If however, your goal is to decrease pain you may want to focus more on long sustained passive stretches that increase the range of motion around a joint. Here's a rundown of the most common forms of stretching and what they're good for, as well as a sample static stretching program.

Static Stretches

This is a passive stretch because it is non-moving, meaning that you just get into a stretch position and hold it. Static stretches also are plastic stretches, which promote more permanent lengthening of the connective tissue. In contrast, elastic stretches (such as ballistic stretches) promote a temporary lengthening of tissue. To perform a static stretch you should exhale as you go into the stretch and then hold the position without bouncing for approximately 20 seconds. Stretch to the point that you feel moderate tension—never pain.

Static stretches should be performed at the end of a cardiovascular workout such as running, biking or aerobics, when your muscles are warm and in the best condition to be lengthened. Since these stretches promote permanent lengthening of the connective tissue around a joint, they are effective at lengthening tight muscles and preventing injury.

Ballistic Stretches

A form of active flexibility training, ballistic stretches prepare the body for high-speed movement. They involve rapid, uncontrolled bouncing movements at a joint. Many movements in sports and exercise are ballistic in nature, so this type of stretching may be useful for explosive power athletes training for the high speed ballistic movements of their sport.

"Ballistic stretching is applied based on what a person is going to do," says Mike. "There is such an overload on joints and muscles that it is more uncontrolled than other active or passive stretches. You leave a comfort zone and enter a range that the body cannot control." The movements should be rhythmic and closely mimic the movement of the sport. Because of its uncontrolled nature, ballistic stretching is not recommended for the general population.

> **Sample ballistic stretch**: To stretch your hamstrings sit with your legs out in front of you. Bend forward from your torso, reach toward your toes and bounce up and down.

PNF Stretches

This is a combination of active and passive stretching. PNF stands for Proprioceptive Neuromuscular Facilitation. These stretches quicken the response of your neuromuscular system (remember that the central nervous systems is at the heart of all movement). Basically, to do a PNF stretch you first perform a five-to ten-second isometric contraction of the muscle and then release the tension, while someone else presses you further into the stretch. PNF stretches increase your mobility as they allow you to take a stretch deeper than is possible with static stretching.

> **Sample PNF stretch:** To stretch your hamstrings lie on your back with one leg up. Another person then places his/her hands underneath your leg and pushes the leg toward your head while you push downward. This creates an isometric contraction in your hamstrings, which you hold for about five to ten seconds. Then, let go, relax and perform a passive hamstring stretch (with your leg relaxed, the other person pushes your leg toward your head).

Active-Isolated Stretches

Active-Isolated Stretching (also known as A-I Stretching) is an active flexibility program that isolates the muscles to be stretched. The principle behind A-I stretch is to fire up or contract the primary muscle (agonist) so that you place the opposing muscle (antagonist) in a state of relaxation. For example, if you wanted to do an A-I stretch for your hamstrings, you would actively contract your quadriceps by lifting your leg up as far as you can from a supine position (lying on your back). At that point intensity is added through use of a prop (such as a towel or tubing) or an assistant, and the stretch is held for one-and-a-half to two seconds before repeating it. Stretches usually are done eight-12 times per muscle. A-I stretches are growing in popularity because they have been found to promote function and healing, and to prevent injury. However, because they are so intense, it is wise to contact a professional trained in A-I stretching or to read up on proper form.

> **Sample A-I stretch:** To stretch your hamstrings you would lie on your back and lift your leg up as far as you can; once you're at that point you use a towel wrapped around your leg to pull your leg further in toward your head for no more than two seconds; then lower the leg and repeat the stretch several times without any rest periods.

Active Warm-up

Although you might not consider slow jogging in place prior to running a form of stretching, it is an active flexibility program that is extremely functional because it specifically prepares you for your workout. "Just a brisk walk prior to a run is a warm-up that increases heart rate, range of motion, and flexibility," notes Mike, who recommends doing an active flexibility warm-up before your main exercise. In essence the active warm-up is simply a reduced-intensity form of your main workout. This gradually gets your body ready to perform at higher intensities.

SAFETY IN STRETCHING

While all these type of stretches have their benefits, you need to bear in mind certain safety issues. First, never stretch to the point where you feel pain. "The body is designed to stretch only to 1.6 times its resting length," explains Mike. Know what a good stretch feels like, as compared to one that may potentially hurt you. Mike recommends using the Borg Scale of Exertion1 to analyze the intensity of your stretch. The scale is based on a 0-10 point range. Once you're in the stretch determine how hard you are working. "0" means you are feeling nothing at all, 5 means you're feeling the stretch pretty intensely, 10 means you feel like you're going to break something. You want to stay in the 4-7 range.

Mike also has some concerns about many of the currently popular activities that require a tremendous amount of flexibility. "Beware of yoga and kickboxing. We're all not built the same and these disciplines require a great deal of flexibility. For example in yoga, you shouldn't feel like you have to be at the same level as the instructor and other people in the class. Never force your body to go into a position," he warns.

SAMPLE STATIC STRETCH PROGRAM

On the next pages you'll find a sample static stretch program you can do seated on a mat. For each of these stretches, slowly exhale as you go into the stretch position, then hold the stretch without bouncing for at least 20 seconds before moving on to the next position. Breathe throughout each stretch, and stretch only to the point of tension or mild discomfort. As you hold the stretch, you should feel the tension begin to subside. You might want to play some soothing music to help you relax into the stretches.

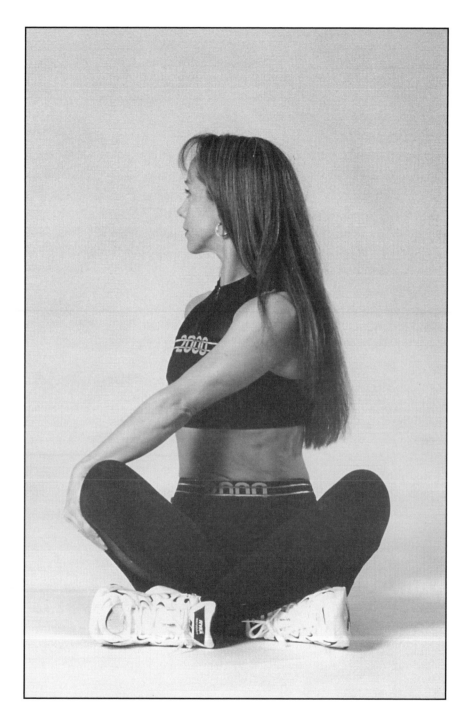

THE SPINAL TWIST

Sit with your legs crossed at your ankles, your back straight and abdominals held in. Place your left hand on your right knee and your right hand behind your right hip. Twist your torso to the right, looking behind you. Hold. Repeat on other side.

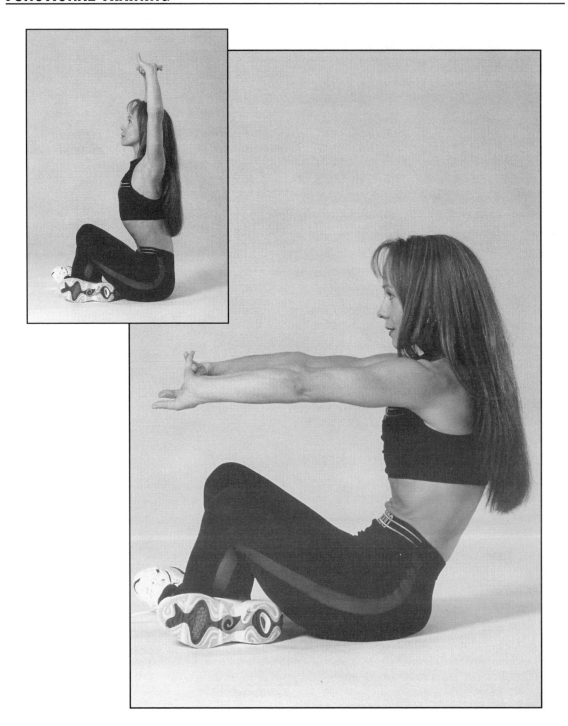

UPPER BACK STRETCH

Lift your arms straight over your head as you inhale. Interlace your fingers. Exhale and bring your arms in front of you, pushing forward as you pull you stomach back (as if you were punched in the stomach). Hold. To increase the intensity of this stretch hold onto a fixed surface such as a doorknob as you pull back.

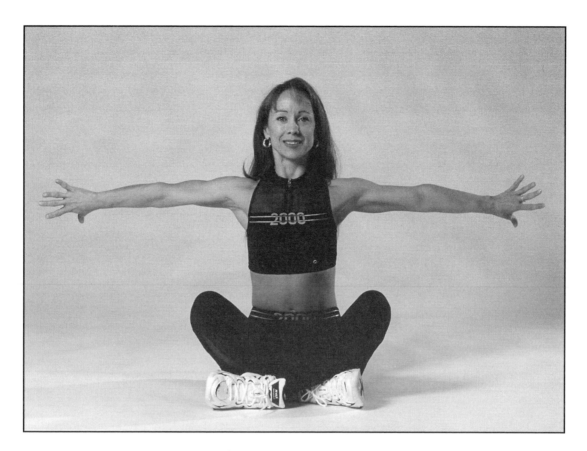

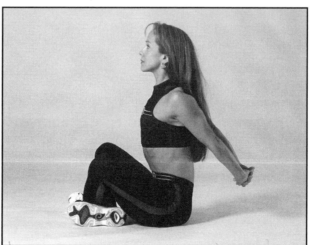

CHEST OPENER

Extend your arms straight out to the side, parallel to the floor and inhale. As you exhale, bring your arms behind your back, interlace your fingers and pull your arms behind your body. Hold.

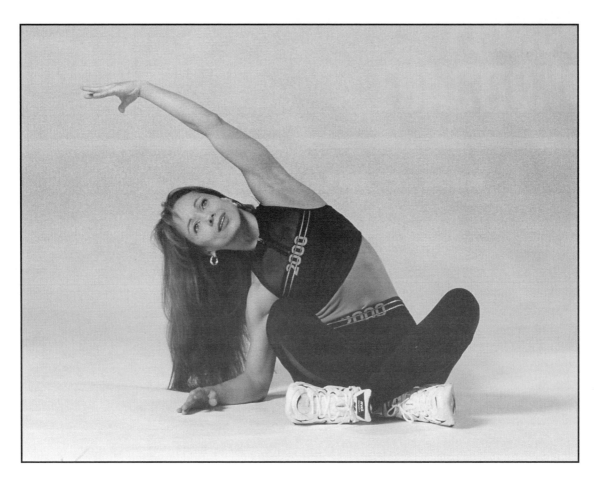

SIDE STRETCH

Place your right forearm or hand down on the mat next to your right leg. Inhale. As you exhale bend over to your right side, with your left arm making an arc over your head. Hold. Repeat on other side.

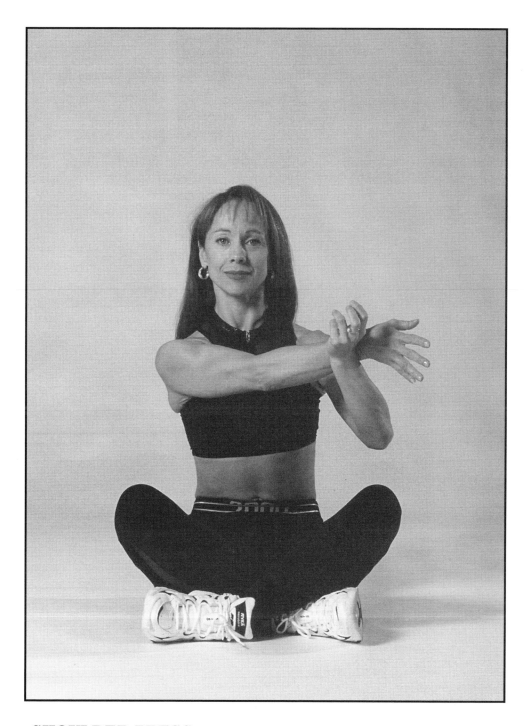

SHOULDER PRESS
Gently pull your right arm across your chest, making sure to keep your right shoulder relaxed (not pressed up to your ear). Apply pressure with your left arm to stretch your right shoulder. Hold. Switch sides.

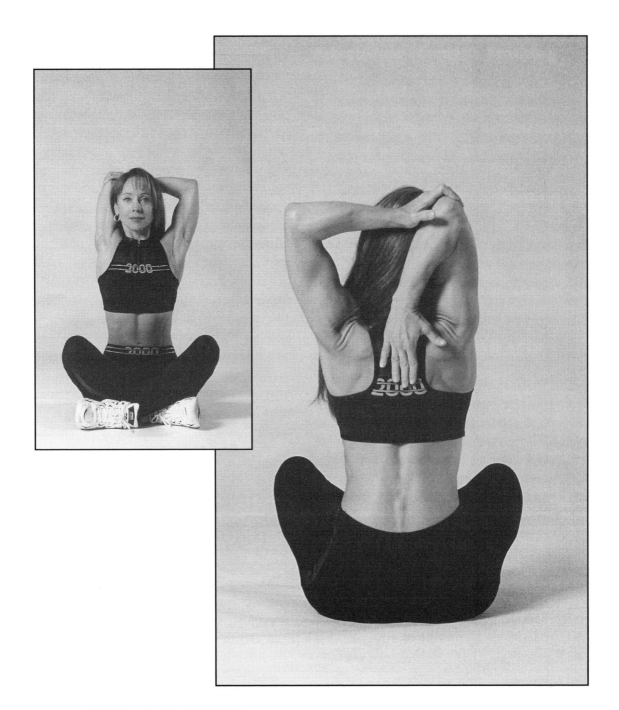

TRICEPS STRETCH

Begin with your right arm extended above your head. Slowly bend that arm, so that your right hand reaches behind your neck and your elbow is overhead. Use your left hand to apply firm but gentle pressure right below your elbow. Hold. Switch arms.

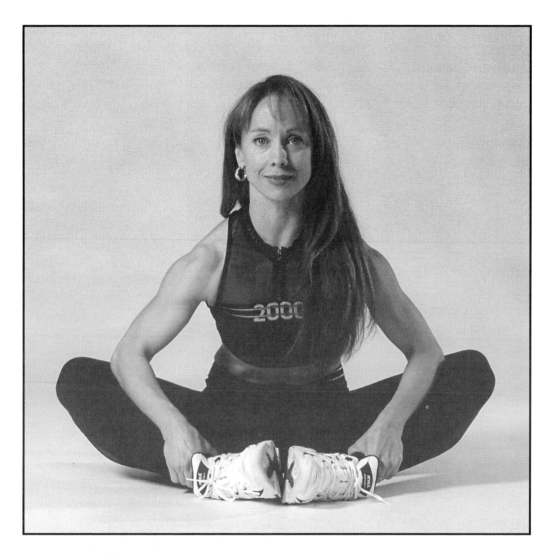

INNER THIGH STRETCH

Sit with the soles of your feet touching. Bring your legs in as close as possible to your body. Bend your arms and exhale as you apply downward pressure with your forearms to stretch your inner thighs.

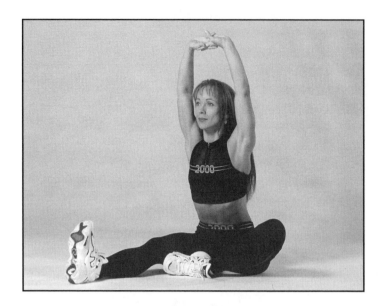

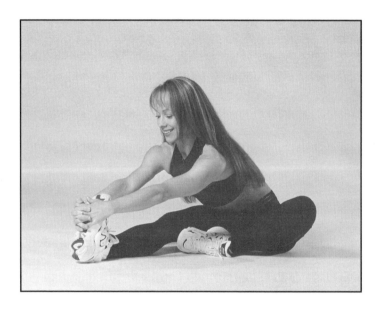

HAMSTRING STRETCH

Sit with your right leg extended out in front of you, and the left bent so that the heel of your left foot is against your right inner thigh. Interlace your fingers and lift your arms overhead as you inhale. Exhale and slowly bring your arms and torso forward, making sure that you initiate the movement from the base of your spine. Go as far forward as you can without feeling pain. Hold. Switch legs.

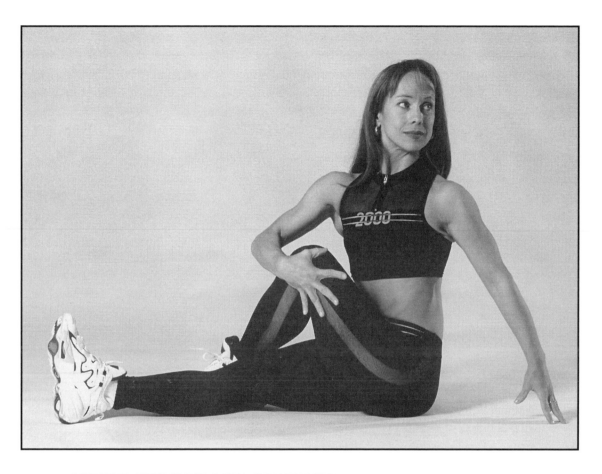

OUTER THIGH/BACK STRETCH

Sit with your right leg extended out in front of you and left leg crossed over. Hook your right arm around your left leg, pressing the left leg close to your chest. Hold. Repeat on other leg.

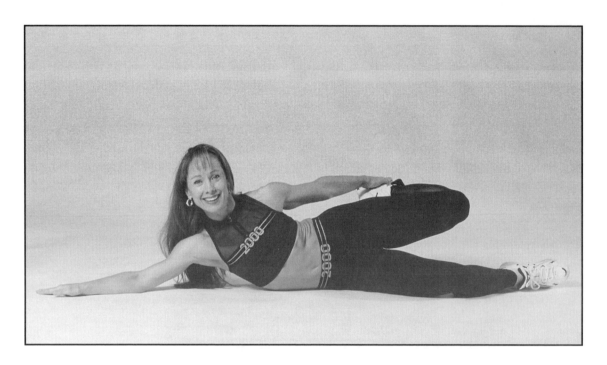

QUADRICEPS STRETCH

Lie on your right side with both legs bent at about 90 degree angles. Hold your left foot with your left hand and pull your left leg behind you until you feel a stretch in the front of your thigh. Hold. Repeat on other side.

HOW BALANCED ARE YOU?

Balance is essential not only to excel in a sport or fitness activity, but also to be able to perform daily life activities. Imagine if we lost our balance every time we got up from a chair. Older adults in particular find that they may begin to lose balance due to diminished vision, diminished reaction time and a tendency to be reactive and tentative, which is part of the aging process. The somatosensory system is what provides information to the brain regarding where your body is in space (e.g. through kinesthetic awareness and proprioception). Defects in this system cause people to encounter problems with balance.

In addition to the older adult, younger people may have no trouble with balance when doing the basic activities of life, but may find that they are challenged when they are doing a more complicated activity or sports move, such as a weighted lunge.

You can see that balance work is a very useful component to add to your training. The sample core training program that Paul Chek provides in the following chapter includes several exercises that work on improving balance, since your body's ability to balance is dependent on the stability and strength of its core muscles. In addition, here are a few other balance-specific exercises for you to try.

(Remember the rule of progression: start with a static surface such as a floor or mat and progress to an unstable one, such as a wobble board or stability ball, and begin trying to balance while not moving; progress to balancing while moving.)

- Shift your weight from having your feet flat on the floor to raising up to the balls of your feet. Then try doing the same thing with both eyes closed.

- Stand and lift your left leg out in front of you; hold it, trying not to wobble. Once you've mastered this, try to balance with your eyes closed. Progress to balancing (eyes open) while moving your leg from in front of you to out to your side to behind you. Finally, do the same exercise with your eyes closed.

- Do squats and pushups on a wobble board.

- Walk on your toes; walk on your heels.

MIKE'S FINAL WORD:

"I have clients who have increased flexibility substantially, usually after about four to six weeks of training. Don't expect changes to occur overnight. I have a client—a middle aged lawyer—who was having trouble with his hip and lower back. After doing active flexibility training he has seen remarkable benefits—decreased pain and increased flexibility. Older adults notice that they can walk better, step off a curb, and that their activity level goes up."

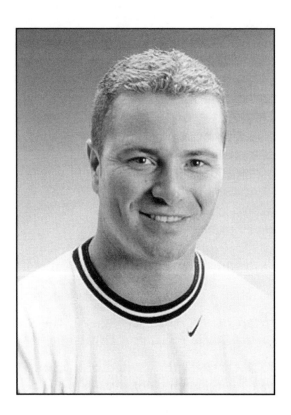

**Michael Jenniex, MA, NSCA, AIFE,
Program Director, Whitaker Wellness Center, Naples, Fla.
Strength Coach, Florida Gulf Coast University
Pro Trainer, Southeast region, Bodytraining Systems**

CHAPTER 4

CORE & STABILITY TRAINING

You've seen them at the gym, and perhaps you are one of them: people breathing heavily through 100 crunches, believing that this is the only way to get a toned stomach, that the more crunches done, the better. If 100 is good, 120 must be better! Right? This chapter, perhaps the most important one in the book, challenges that belief.

WHAT DOES TRAINING YOUR BODY'S CORE MEAN?

Many people think of the core as the abdominals, so they do a lot of abdominal exercises and think they have gained strength in their centers. This approach, however, is incomplete. Your core is the entire midsection of your body including not only the abdominals, but the lower back and pelvis as well, and the entire core (both inner and outer) must be worked. The importance of having a strong core cannot be overemphasized, because just as the heart is your body's great blood pump, the core is your body's great energy pump, or as Paul Chek puts it, "the force conductor," behind all of our movements.

Paul knows a lot about core training. An internationally acclaimed speaker and consultant, Chek (MMS, NMT, HHP) draws upon 16 years of experience in corrective and high performance exercise kinesiology. He is the author of over 50 videos, books, seminars and correspondence courses. In addition, he is founder of the C.H.E.K. Institute in California-an educational organization that certifies advanced exercise specialists with a Corrective High-Performance Exercise Kinesiology Certification. These credentials highlight Paul's important role as an expert who brings the results of scientific research into practice.

Paul's passion about functional and core training is evident in his strong, sometimes aggressive opinions about what he considers functional and what is dangerous, and what is good core training versus bad core training. In fact, his depth of experience in the field—years spent working in rehabilitation, strength and conditioning have provided him with a "say it like it is" approach. For example, he's been known to declare the following: "Machine training in general is suitable for only two groups of human beings; body builders and the near dead!" One thing for sure, you can count on Paul to call it as he sees it!

In this chapter, Paul provides his perspective on functional training in general, an overview of core training including the core's function, and the wrong and right ways to train your core. At the end of the chapter you will find some sample balance and core exercises from his book *The Golf Biomechanics Manual (1999)*.

CHEK GUIDELINES OF FUNCTIONAL TRAINING:

WHAT TO LOOK FOR

According to Paul, to determine if what you are doing is truly functional training, you need to answer the following question: Are your training programs living up to the meaning of the term 'functional': are they useful and applicable, something that serves the purpose for which they were designed?

The C.H.E.K. Institute uses several guidelines to prescribe exercises that are functional. These are rather technical and will not be expanded upon much here, but to give you a sense of the characteristic components of functional exercise, they are listed below, taken from an article written by Paul for the website *Personal Training on the Net*, a site that contains the latest articles in exercise research by renowned fitness professionals. (If you would like to read Paul's complete article "What is Functional Exercise" go to the website PTontheNet.com).[1]

CHARACTERISTICS OF FUNCTIONAL EXERCISE

1. **Works on your righting and equilibrium reflexes** (for example, being able to restore balance to prevent a fall).

2. **Helps to maintain your center of gravity over your base of support** (i.e. your balance).

3. **Based on generalized motor program compatibility** (Your brain recognizes movement patterns that are similar and stores them as a generalized motor program. In practical terms, doing squats with resistance will improve your jumping ability because the movement patterns of a squat and a jump are so close).

4. **Open vs. closed chain exercise** (If you recall, open chain exercises are those in which the end of the movement is not fixed and closed chain exercises are those in which the end of the movement is against a fixed surface that cannot be moved. Try to choose exercises that resemble the actual environment to which you want to apply them. For example, if you want to improve your rock climbing ability, doing lat pull downs for your upper body strength will do little to help you since in this open chain exercise you must pull the load (the bar) toward you, which is not what you do on a rock. Instead, do chin-ups (a closed chain exercise) in which you must pull your

body up past your fixed hand, which more closely resembles what you would do when rock climbing).

5. **Improves your ability to move,** including strength, power, endurance, flexibility, agility, balance and coordination.

6. **Moves from muscular isolation to integration.** Functional training is about integrating muscles, doing compound exercises instead of ones that isolate muscles (Paul goes into this in detail in his foreword).

WHAT TO WATCH OUT FOR

IMPROPER RESISTANCE AND FORM

Unfortunately, Paul has seen a lot that gets promoted as "functional exercise" in gyms, on videos, and in articles that he believes in fact, can be downright dangerous. "One of my primary concerns with what's going on today is that there is a group of leaders who have taken the concept of functional exercise to a bit of an extreme," he explains. "For example, I've seen articles that show people doing lunges with a rounded back and forward reaching arms, whether they be holding a medicine ball or a weight in their hands, under the premise that when you are using a tennis racket that your spine is rounded and that's the natural position to be in." (He was once approached in New Zealand as a consultant by someone who was doing lunges with 225 pounds and rounding his back because he was told that it was functional.) The problem with this line of reasoning Paul explains, is that people are exposed to exercises with very high levels of resistance that *do not match the resistance of the sport or activity they want to excel in.*

"When people have the interpretation that function in the gym equates to function on the field there can be significant problems. When you're talking about swinging a tennis racket that may weigh less than one pound, you're talking about a very light object," Paul says.

He also notes that in a sports situation, whether it be tennis or baseball or golf, *you rarely ever perform the exact same movement with the exact same load twice.* "It's extremely rare that the same tissues (ligaments, joint capsules, muscles, or even bony structures) ever get loaded the same way twice in a row. However, when you take someone into a gym environment and you put them on a cable machine or put a barbell across their back, or give them a medicine ball, you're often exposing them repetitiously week after week to high speed with a high resistance load that can potentially damage tissues. We have to look at the concepts of what truly is functional exercise, because doing this can easily cause injury, which becomes dysfunctional exercise in my opinion," Paul says.

GROUP TRAINING CLASSES

Another caveat of Paul's has to do with group functional training exercise classes, such as boot camp training and plyometric sports conditioning classes. While many people swear by them and such classes are in fact very popular, Paul's concern is that with a large group of people it is very difficult for an instructor or trainer to ensure that each person is working at the appropriate level and in a way that follows that all important "P" word—progression. In fact, Paul likens such classes to a mass drug prescription. "You give everyone the same drug (or exercise): ten people do great, ten die, and ten don't know what the hell's going on."

He notes certain power exercise training programs, such as kickboxing, which are extremely intense and require a certain baseline level of fitness before they can be taken safely. Yet these higher-level classes often are full of beginning exercisers or deconditioned people who are excited by the latest trend. Consequently, they end up doing movements like high kicks and fast jumps, for which their bodies are not prepared. They don't have the necessary core strength or flexibility and haven't built up to the level of fitness required to safely do power training.

"When you expose people to the wrong progression, you get tricked by changes in aesthetics or momentary results, but the long-range result is always mechanical breakdown and ultimately, an increased risk of drop out," says Paul. He teaches that the body must be developed according to a basic progression formula:

- Restore flexibility and muscle balance
- Improve joint stability
- Move on to strength training
- Only after a base conditioning phase of strength training should you try power type exercises.

GETTING TO THE CORE

Definitions of which parts of your body constitute the core may differ to a degree, depending upon whom you ask. Textbooks define the area essentially as the rib cage and spine, but Paul likes to include the head and neck as well. He believes that leaving out these parts compartmentalizes the body, and you know that the major message of this book is that the body does not function in separate parts.

All right, given that the core is made up of your pelvis, abdominals, entire spine, as well as your head and your neck, what's so important about it? What does it do? A lot. It:

- Protects your internal organs, spinal cord and nervous system.
- Circulates blood and lymph throughout your body.
- Serves as a system for stabilizing and moving your body.
- Acts as a bridge between your arms and legs.

"No matter how you slice it, your core is pretty much the key region of your body," says Paul. "In any sport or work environment, the core actually serves as a force conductor or transmitter to take the force from the legs and transfer it through the core into the arms." He notes the false impression many of us have that our legs and arms carry our body's core along and that the spine is a passive column. In fact, the core and spine are the engines that drive all of our movement.

WHY TRAIN THE CORE?

Functional training essentially begins at your body's core. If we don't have strong centers, there is little that we will be able to do in this world. Unfortunately, this is an area of the body that has been neglected both in traditional training and by the way we modern humans live.

Paul notes that core training is particularly important in today's sedentary environment, where you don't have to get up to do much of anything for most of the day. "We've gone from an existence of high level athletic demand, to an existence where people can sit behind a computer all day long and never move. Think about how many times you've seen someone driving around a mall for half an hour trying to find a spot so they can save themselves 30 seconds of walking." The problem is that we are seeing injuries that result from this lack of use. Because when these people do have to move—whether to do a chore or carry a baby—they find that they don't have the necessary strength and are highly prone to back injuries.

Core training that strengthens the vital muscles of your body's center is essential then not only to improve your athletic performance, but also to avoid serious injury that may become chronic and severely affect the quality of your life. In fact, the American College of Sports Medicine's *Health & Fitness Journal* recently reported that lower back injury is the second most common health problem in the United States, with back pain second only to childbirth for sending people to the hospital.[2]

TRAINING THE CORE

WHAT'S WRONG

Here's the sticky point. Despite all the attention giving to abdominal training in gyms, on videos and in physical education classes, little is actually of use in strengthening your core. "The kind of core training being done today unfortunately is not making anything better; it's making it worse," says Paul.

WHAT'S GOING ON?

As Paul explains, the most common exercises being used worldwide and on teams of all types for abdominal training are things such as crunches, sit ups, reverse crunches and hanging leg raises. Wait a minute! What's wrong with a crunch? "Laying on the floor and doing crunches only tightens the rectus abdominis and the anterior portion of the external oblique," he says. In other words, you are only working the outer core muscles. These outer muscles are dependent on the muscles of the inner core (such as the transverse abdominis and multifidious) for stabilization. Your body must be stabilized in order to be able to effectively and safely generate the force needed for any activity.

Paul uses a pirate ship analogy to help illustrate this point, likening the ship's mast to a human vertebral column: remember that in this case the human vertebral column (mast) has 24 mobile segments! If the segments are not stabilized by the smaller, inner muscles and you continue to tighten the "guy wires" (or outer core muscles) over and over again without proportion to the same amount of work required to stabilize the core, you will collapse the mast.

In addition to focusing too much on outer unit training, Paul finds a lot of imbalance in terms of the planes in which people do abdominal work, with most people doing much more flexion than extension, very little left-to-right work, and not enough rotation. "We're perpetuating spinal dysfunction by shortening the muscles that pull our bodies into the very position that gravity will put you in if your postural muscles get weak." Think about it. Doing a basic crunch depresses or lowers your chest, pulls your head and shoulders forward and flattens your back. This "pulling down and forward" action is doing nothing to help you fight gravity or to have a body that can function optimally in a multi-dimensional environment. In addition, your lower back muscles are probably weak and in imbalance with an overly trained outer core.

WHAT'S RIGHT

So throw out all the curls, reverse crunches and twists? Not entirely, but you need to make sure that you *first* pay attention to your inner core muscles, and give them the focus they deserve because if you are like most people, you've spent way too much time on your outer muscles and are suffering from muscular imbalance.

Paul recommends a balanced exercise program that strengthens the inner unit so that it can handle the outer unit and then to develop the two together. "People have to remember that core conditioning is movement pattern specific. The world's greatest cruncher may not be able to push the food cart down the aisle of the airplane because laying on the ground is so distinctly different from pushing a cart that the brain can't take that crunch exercise and say, 'I'm going to use that crunch exercise to push this cart better,'" he explains. Bringing it back to the pirate ship analogy, you're tightening guy wires and not tightening the rest of the wires proportionately; when the heavy cart comes to an abrupt stop your brain cannot go from the crunch exercise you did on the floor to a standing activity where it has to stabilize every joint in the body in a split second.

To bring your body back into balance you need first to focus core training on the inner core muscles (because these are the parts of our system that are not working). When you do crunches and twists from a lying down position you are focusing on the frontal outer muscles, which are the rectus abdominis and the external obliques. What you want to focus on are the inner muscles that stabilize your whole body: the diaphragm, the multifidious (deep stabilizer muscles of your back), the pelvic floor muscles and the transverse abdominis muscle.

Paul recommends that you first consult a knowledgeable fitness professional who can assess the function of your inner core muscles. His website, chekinstitute.com, lists and locates all people trained by the C.H.E.K. Institute. You can also pick up Paul's new book *Flatten Your Abs Forever* (due out in 2001) in which he demonstrates how to assess the function of your inner core so you can restore and build your way to strong, sleek abdominals and true core strength.

So, first you need to isolate the problem areas and work on them, giving your outer core muscles a rest until the inner core muscles catch up. Once you've corrected the imbalance you need to learn how to use your core in the movement patterns (meaning while you are in motion) that are most common in sports and in daily life. After all, in daily life we don't need to do crunches, but we do need to do things like kneel, push open a heavy door while walking or balance on one leg when reaching up to retrieve an object from a top shelf. And in sports we need to twist, bend and move fast all within a very short time frame, requiring balance and stability.

Paul has developed what he calls the Primal Pattern™ system of movement, which is a quick and effective way to analyze movement to determine which patterns need work. The seven primary movement patterns are squatting, lunging, bending, pushing, pulling, twisting and gait (walking, jogging and running). If you have trouble squatting it may very well be because your inner abdominals, in particular the transverse abdominis, are too weak, because the transverse abdominis is a primary stabilizing muscle when you do a squat. If this is the case, then you need to first do isolation work for your transverse abdominals; then once they have gotten stronger, you need to do squatting, perhaps first against a stability ball, then on your own; and then with dumbbells or while holding a medicine ball to your chest.

Remember, virtually everything you do in the standing position is really a core exercise, since your core needs to work to stabilize your body so that it has a solid foundation from which you can move. "Every time you do a lunge, or grab the handle of the cable machine with one hand you are doing a core exercise," says Paul. Because you can work the core in so many different ways, depending on the movement pattern used, you can do core training every day.

In addition to incorporating exercises that develop the stabilizer muscles of the core and using the core in movement patterns, Paul recommends getting off the machines and doing your weight training with free weights, tubing or cables. Again: Integrate, don't isolate! If you have an addiction to machines, start your training program with functional exercise. After you have trained two to three functional movements, finish training with some traditional bodybuilding exercises. At least that way you will be able to *move as good as you look*!

On the following pages you will find sample exercises that work your core muscles, which have been reprinted with permission, from Paul's book *The Golf Biomechanics Manual*. These exercises follow a specific progression (Paul calls them phases), going from building initial strength in the core to more advanced exercises that incorporate movement. See how different they are from all those crunches you've been doing!

These are just a sampling of the types of core exercises you can do and include representative exercises from the first three phases of Paul's seven-phase strengthening program.

Try these exercises to help develop a strong stable core. Be sure to master the early phase exercises first before progressing to more difficult ones. A note about the exercises: Reps refers to the number of exercises you will do in each set. After doing the number of reps indicated, rest allowing your body to adapt, and then perform the next set. Also it is essential that you only do as many exercises as you can in perfect form. Watch yourself in a mirror or use a spotter if possible to ensure that your form is good.

THE IMPORTANCE OF CORE TRAINING

Fitness Expert Paul Chek relates the following example illustrating the importance of core training:

"I rehab many injured flight attendants who push food trolleys up and down the aisle and maybe hit rough turbulence and accidentally bang into a seat, causing the cart to stop abruptly. What happens is that they are generating the force to move the cart with their legs, but in order to move the cart the core has to serve as the bridge mechanism to get the force of their legs off the floor of the aircraft and up into their arms to actually push the cart. If these attendants spend time doing a lot of isolated training of their arms and legs, and have poor core function, then the instant that the cart stops, the force cannot be effectively dissipated through their bodies. Wherever there is a dysfunction of the core, there will be a blockage of energy transfer, which usually is in the lumbar spine and produces back injuries."

PAUL CHEK'S CORE TRAINING PROGRAM PHASE I

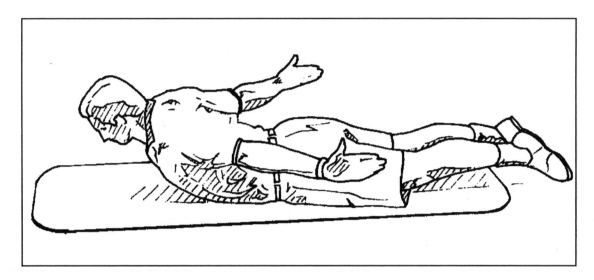

PRONE COBRA

Lie face down on a mat or carpet. Squeeze your shoulder blades together and turn your shoulders out as you lift your torso. Palms should face away from your body. Keep your head and neck in alignment and your toes touching the floor. Hold the position for 30 seconds; rest 15 seconds. Perform 1-8 reps and 1-2 sets. The Cobra conditions your postural muscles.

VERTICAL HORSE STANCE

Start on your hands and knees, with your shoulders directly above your wrists and your hips above your knees. Ideally, you should place a straight rod along your spine to hold perfect spinal alignment; the rod should be parallel to the floor (the best is a wooden closet rod 6 ' x 1 3/8").

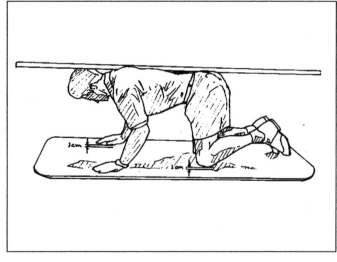

Draw your navel up and inward toward your spine to create a space between your belt and your stomach. Lift one hand off the floor just enough to slide a sheet of paper between your hand and the floor. Then, lift the opposite knee to the same height. Keep the rod level. Hold the position for 10 seconds; then switch hands and knees. Perform 1-3 sets of 10 reps. The vertical horse stance improves control and strength of key stabilizer muscles.

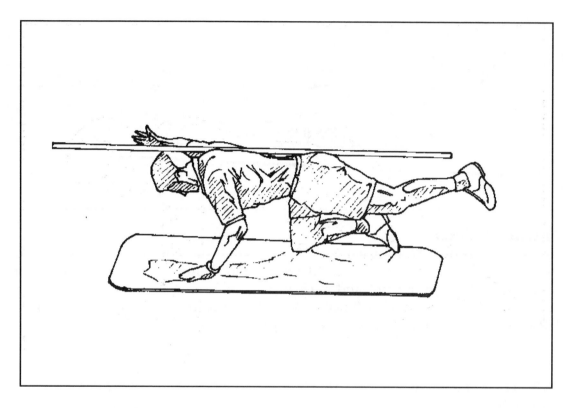

HORIZONTAL HORSE STANCE

Start from the same position as for the vertical horse stance. Raise one arm to 4 degrees off the midline of your body, holding it in the same plane as the midline of your body. Lift your opposite leg—without tilting your pelvis forward—and hold your leg out straight. Do not allow your shoulders or pelvis to lose their horizontal relationship with the floor. Hold this position for 10 seconds; then switch sides. Perform 1-3 sets of 10 reps. The horizontal horse stance also improves control and strength of key stabilizer muscles.

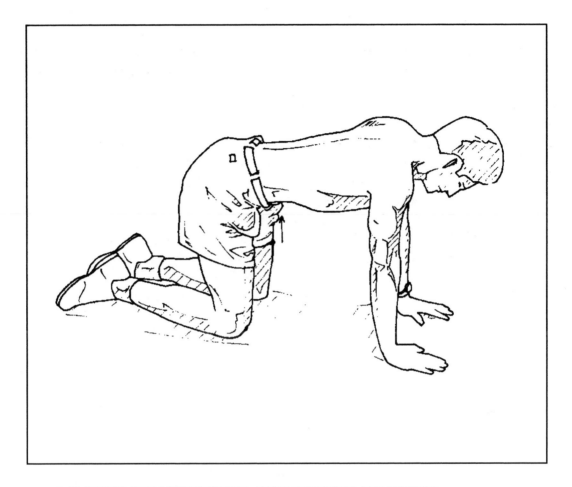

4 POINT TRANSVERSE ABDOMINIS TRAINER

Start on your hands and your knees, with your spine in neutral alignment, inhale deeply and allow your belly to drop toward the floor. Exhale and draw your navel in toward your spine as far as you can. Hold that position for 10 seconds, or as long as you can comfortably without taking a breath (up to 10 seconds). Perform 1 to 3 sets of 10 repetitions. This is a great exercise to strengthen the all-important transverse abdominal muscles.

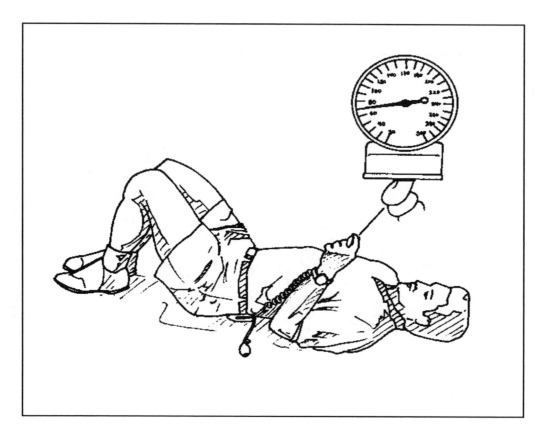

LOWER ABDOMINAL EXERCISE

(For this exercise you need to use a blood pressure cuff with an extender hose to properly gauge the intensity of your work. Place the blood pressure cuff (BPC) under your lower back, behind your navel. Lie down with your knees bent and feet flat and pump the BPC up to 40 mm Hg.

Exhale and draw your navel inward toward your spine as you gently tilt the pelvis forward. The BPC (now compressed) should read a higher level of pressure (eg. 70 mm Hg.); or you can simply try holding the pressure at 40mmHg while moving your legs in the beginning. Relax your entire body as you try to hold the higher intensity level for 10 seconds. Perform 1-3 sets of 10 repetitions. DO NOT HOLD YOUR BREATH. Then rest for ten seconds. This helps to stabilize your spine and your whole musculoskeletal system.

Superman
Hip ext no arms

PHASE II

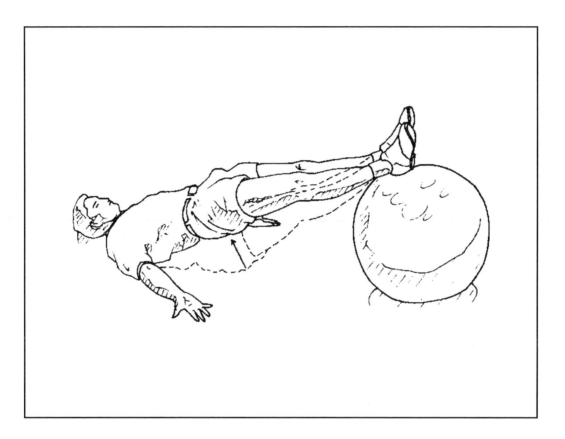

SUPINE HIP EXTENSION
Lie on your back with your feet on the ball. Start with your feet wide and narrow them as you get stronger. Put your arms out to the side, palms facing up. From the start position, extend your hips into the air on a count of three until you line up your ankle, hip and shoulder. Hold for three seconds, then lower for three seconds. Perform 1-3 sets of 8-12 reps. A

As you get stronger, move your hands closer to your body. Progress to the point where you can do the exercise with your arms across your chest and your heels only on the ball. This is an excellent exercise that conditions your core muscles, as well as trains your hamstrings, gluteals and back to work together, and improves balance, coordination and postural endurance.

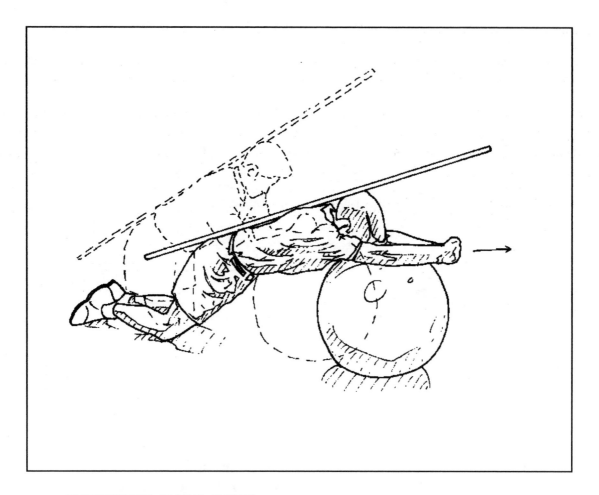

FORWARD BALL ROLL

Kneel in front of the ball, placing your forearms on the ball, with your palms facing each other. If you have a dowel rod, place it on your back. Take a deep breath and pull your navel in toward your spine to slim out your waist slightly. Begin to roll forward moving equally from your hips and shoulders. Stop when you feel you are about to lose spinal alignment. You will know if you are losing alignment if the curves in your spine increase and the stick starts to fall off. Take three seconds to roll forward, hold for three seconds and then roll backwards for three seconds. Perform 1-3 sets of 8-12 reps. This exercise strengthens the abdominals, hip flexors and shoulder extensors.

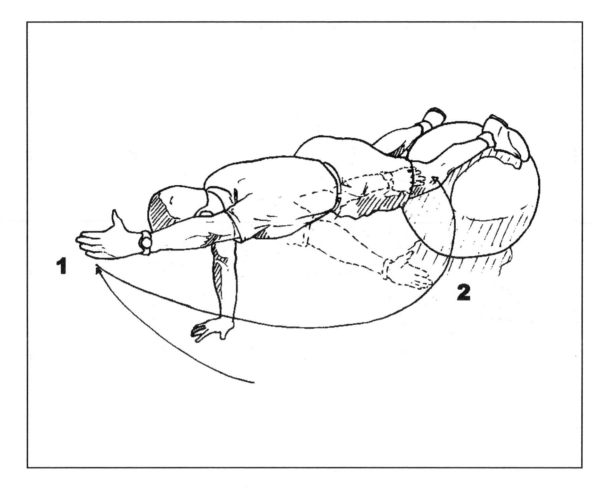

PRONE BRIDGE

This one is particularly challenging, so make sure you do this over a soft surface such as a mat, grass or carpet. Grasp the ball between your shins and assume a pushup position. Hold your body in perfect alignment. When you feel balanced, take one hand off the ground for just a second. As you improve, begin raising the arm forward. Once you can hold your arm out in front of you, begin to move it from the front position in an arc from over your head to your side and back to the floor. Alternate arms. Do 1-3 sets of as many as you can in good form. This exercise strengthens your stabilizers.

PHASE III

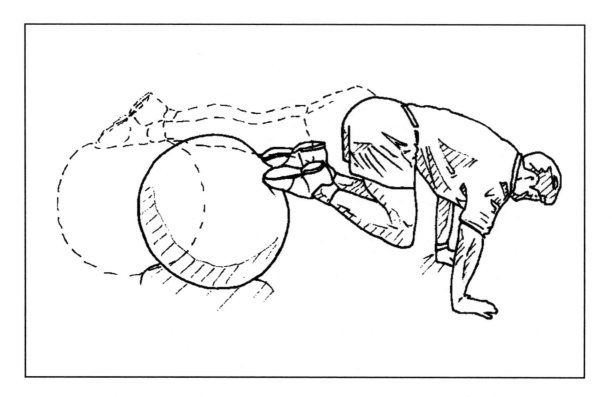

PRONE JACK KNIFE

Begin in a push-up position with your feet on the ball, hands on the ground. Hold your spine straight, with your head and neck in alignment. Draw your legs under your body over a count of two and then return to the start position over a count of two. Perform 1-3 sets of 8-12 repetitions. If the exercise is too hard for you, place more of your leg on the ball. *This exercise strengthens your abdominal muscles a well as your hip flexors and shoulders.*

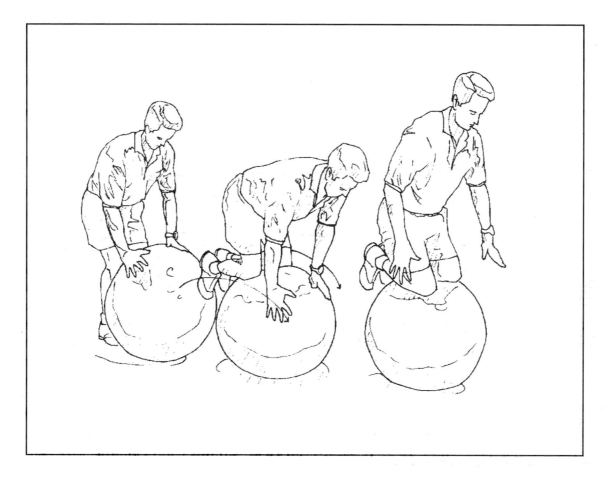

KNEEL ON THE BALL

Place your hands and knees on the ball and slowly rock forward until you are balancing on the ball. From there, let go with your hands and raise up onto your knees. Use as much of your shins as possible to balance and hold onto the ball with your feet for added stability. Kneel for as long as you can without falling off the ball. Perform 4-8 sets of 1-3 reps. This exercise improves balance and coordination.

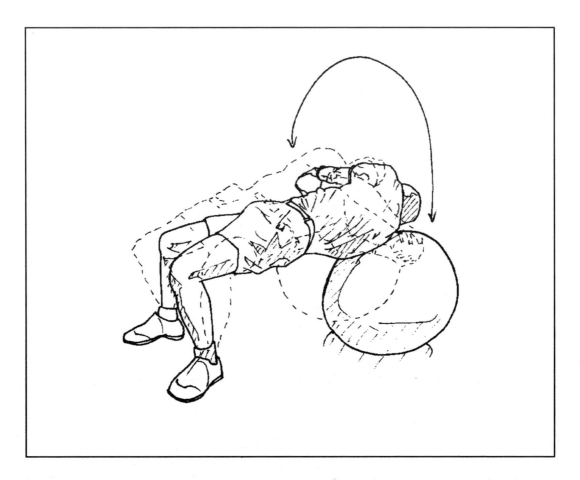

SUPINE RUSSIAN TWIST

Place your back and head on the ball so that your head is supported and your shoulders are across the apex of the ball. Lift your hips so that they are in line with your knees and shoulders. Reach forward and clasp your hands together. Place your tongue on the roof of your mouth to increase activation of your neck flexors, which stabilize your head and neck. Begin to rotate your trunk as far as possible to one side and then to the other using a slow tempo. Progressively increase your range of motion. After about six reps you can speed up to a moderate tempo. Be sure to keep your hips up as you rotate your arms and trunk side to side. Emphasize the trunk rotation. Perform 1-3 sets of 6-10 reps. As you get stronger you can hold a small medicine ball (1-6 pounds) as you perform the rotations. The Supine Russian Twist develops core strength as well as strengthens your pelvic girdle.

PUTTING IT ALL TO WORK FOR YOU!

Now that you have developed both isolated and integrated core strength and control, try applying your new strength and coordination to all your activities of daily living or recreational sports. To do this, simply draw your navel inward slightly and tie a kite string around your waist.

Any time you bend, twist, lift or perform any of the Primal Pattern™ movements, make sure that you start the movement by drawing your navel inward, gently reducing the tension on the string. Start by using this technique with light resistances (you should be able to perform at least 20 repetitions). Once you find that you no longer have to think about activating your deep abdominal wall (core stabilizers) and they are working automatically for you, you can begin performing all your exercises with both greater resistance, *and greater assurance that your body is working correctly!*

TRASH THE WEIGHT BELT

Think the weight belt you wear when lifting is helping to protect your back and make your exercise more efficient? Not according to Paul. Below, he explains why wearing the belt may be doing you and your core more harm than good:

"The weight belt is a false form of support. It creates hoop tension and intra abdominal pressure, adding a false stability to your body. When you do this, the body can sense that there is some stability being created and it will regulate the need for the recruitment of your own inner unit muscles to provide stability.

"The body also is a sensory motor system. If you put a belt around someone, pressure is created on the outer part of your abdominal wall. Your brain always focuses on what's touching the body, so the brain wants to push into the belt, which means that you have to turn on your outer unit muscles which expand the torso to push into the belt (as opposed to turning on the inner unit muscles, which pull your navel inward toward your spine). So the brain begins to learn that it doesn't need to use the inner core muscles, and you end up developing sensory motor amnesia due to lack of use." Result? A weaker inner core!

"I use a number of Paul's techniques and philosophies in my daily training programs and I believe Paul to be the leader in his field of expertise. His ability to teach and encourage proactive thinking and the use of functional principles relating to preventative techniques, injury treatment and rehabilitation is second to none."

—Paul Hamson, Strength & Conditioning Coach, Super League Canberra Raiders

"My hip has not felt this good for over 40 years, and the rest of me was sore but inspired. Paul, you clearly are a genius at what you do, and your forward thinking, and outstanding, functional theories are exciting for all-athletes and non-athletes alike. I wish I had known of you during my competitive years."

—Bob Wall, co-star in Bruce Lee's "Enter The Dragon" Wall Street Properties Realtors

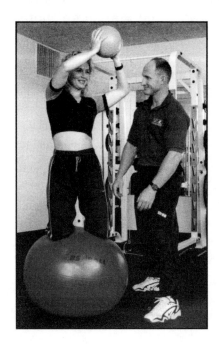

PAUL'S FINAL WORD:

"So many people have been influenced by the machine industry, and they've exercised and built big muscles in the absence of the inner core unit or stabilizing function of any of the working joints. We're coming out of the bodybuilding era, which used to be based on real weight training and integrated function of the body. But bodybuilding has gone from being free weight training to machine training which cannot be applied to standing functional movement."

Paul Chek, MMS, NMT, HHP
Founder, C.H.E.K. Institute
San Diego, Calif.
Tel: 1-800-552-8789
E-mail: info@chekinstitute.com
Website: paulchekseminars.com

CHAPTER 5

ACTIVITIES FOR DAILY LIFE

In spite of all the assistance offered by technology, human beings have not yet reached the day when we can do everything we need to without getting up from the couch or chair (thank God). Even if you are not a regular exerciser you undoubtedly have to walk, bend, get in and out of a car, occasionally lift boxes or packages, or perhaps a small child—and sometimes may even be forced to sprint for a bus or train. Functional training can prepare you to better perform all the physical tasks involved in everyday life in such a way that reduces your risk of injury and increases the ease with which you can do them.

The most common types of everyday-life movements and some examples of those movements are:

Pushing and Pulling: opening a heavy door, pushing a stroller or shopping cart and moving furniture.

Getting Up and Going Down: getting in and out of a car or chair and climbing stairs.

Reaching and Lifting: picking up boxes, putting items on a high shelf and painting a room.

Carrying: carrying groceries, children.

Gripping: opening cans or lids and using tools.

Mobility: walking, running and balancing in many directions.

Personal Trainer Annette Lang, who is the national program director for the Esquerre Fitness Group and an educator for Reebok University, uses functional training with her clients to help them with these movements of daily life. She customizes each program for the individual client after taking into account her client's age and health, and doing a complete assessment of body fat, strength and flexibility levels, cardiovascular fitness and balance. Her clients range from healthy young people to senior citizens.

Annette finds that her biggest challenge lies in getting her clients to make the connection between what they do in the gym to how they should move in daily life. She gives the example:

"As part of our session I have my client do squats, in which she very carefully goes down and lifts up, bending at the knees, keeping the natural curve in her lower back—her form is perfect. Then, when she is finished doing the exercise she bends forward the wrong way to put the weight down! She hasn't made the important connection between her workout and the correct way to move in real life. So my efforts need to be stronger in getting the message across."

Annette loves nothing better than when her clients make that connection, when they come back to tell her that they really think about what they have learned from her when they are working in their garden, moving furniture or riding their bikes. Others say they are no longer uncomfortable at work or in their car, and she often hears statements like, "Wow, I didn't even think about the fact that my back doesn't cramp so much anymore!"

Even if you consider yourself an active person, it is worth your while to review the program in this chapter because of the law of specificity-that in order to truly make your performance in a given task successful, your exercises must be near exact matches to whatever physical activity you want to perform. So, even an ultra marathoner is at risk for back injury when moving furniture if he or she has not done exercises that work the muscles involved in lifting and pushing in the same ways that they are involved when you actually push or lift something.

Likewise, if you are an older adult or sedentary person you will find Annette's program a great starting point on your journey to fitness.

WORKOUT FOR DAILY LIFE ACTIVITIES

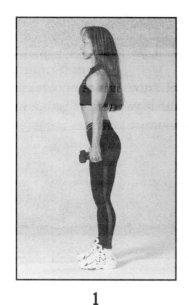

1

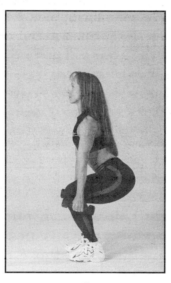

2

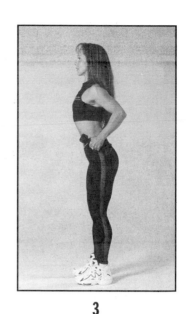

3

SQUATS WITH ROWS

These can be done in the gym using cables or free weights, or at home with free weights. If you don't have weights use a box of books: Hold the weights in your hands. Stand with your feet approximately shoulder width apart or wider; then keeping your knees in line with your toes, bend your legs so that you are sitting down in an imaginary chair. Make sure you keep the natural curve in your lower back and that your abdominals are pulled in tight. As you stand, slowly pull the weights behind you, as if you are doing a rowing movement. Repeat 10-15 times. "This exercise," says Annette, "mimics the proper way to pick something up in real life."

Related Daily Life Movements: getting up/down, pulling, and lifting.

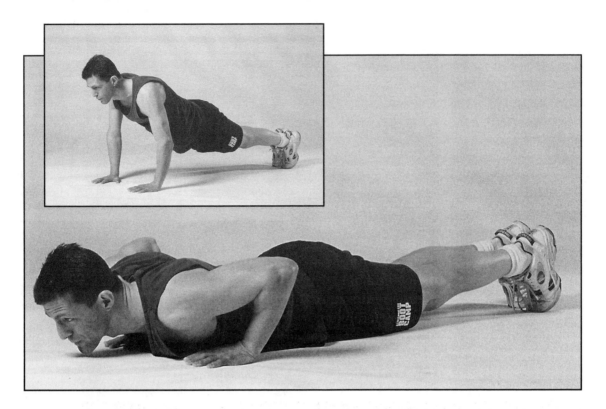

BASIC PUSH-UP

If you have a stability ball you can put either your legs or arms on the ball to address more issues of stability and balance, and do your push-up from those positions. Otherwise, the basic push-up should be done this way: either on your knees (if you're just starting and don't have much strength in your core) or on your toes, with your hands in contact with the floor, at chest level. Bend your arms, lowering your chest as close as possible to the floor while maintaining a flat back, and tight abdominals. Then, push your body away from the floor as you straighten your arms. Repeat 10-15 times.

Variations of this classic functional exercise include making the exercise more powerful by literally pushing hard away from the floor, to force your body to slow the movement down as you hit the floor. Another thing to try is a walking pushup. This exercise, similar to the basic push-up, involves getting into the push-up position and then walking with your hands, back and forth for one or two steps.

Related Daily Life Movement: Pushing.

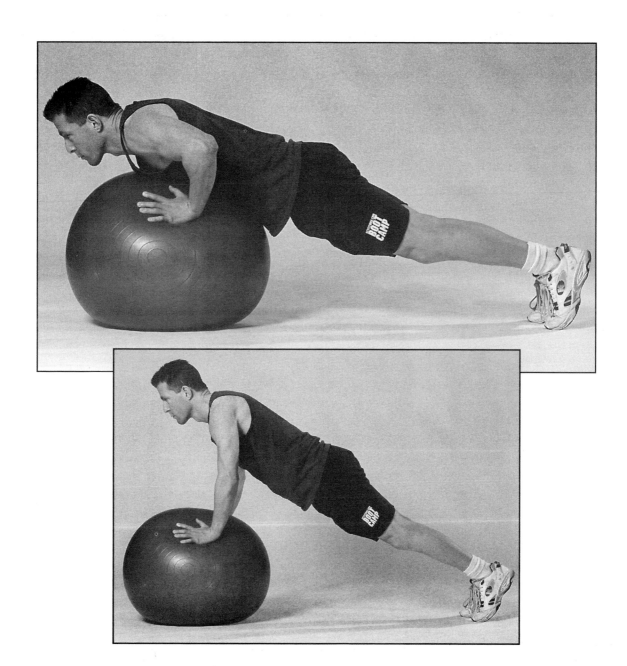

STABILITY BALL PUSH-UP
Perform push-up with hands on a stability ball.

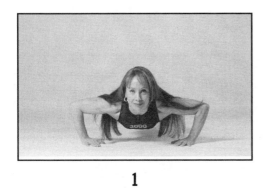

1

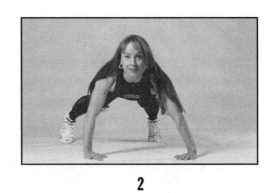

2

3

4

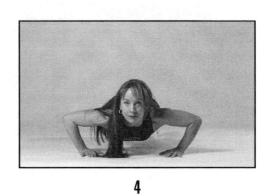

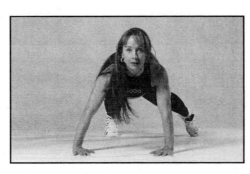

5

THE WALKING PUSH-UP

In push-up position, walk your arms and legs back and forth.

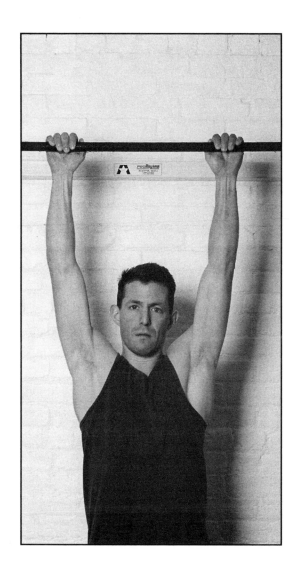
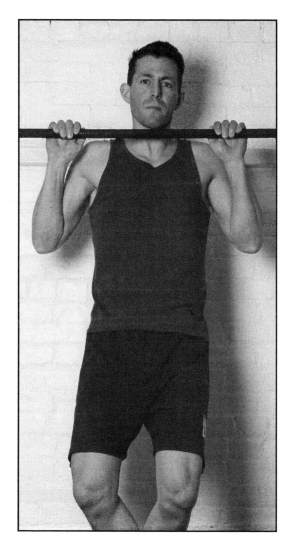

PULL-UPS

Hold onto the bar, hands shoulder-width apart, palms facing away. Pull yourself up until your head is over the bar, then return to starting position. If you can't pull yourself up, jump or use a chair to help get your head over the bar and then concentrate on letting yourself down slowly. This method of working is called "negative" work, which means that you are concentrating on the eccentric, or elongating phase of a muscle contraction when your muscles are lengthening.

Related Daily Life Movement: Pulling and hoisting.

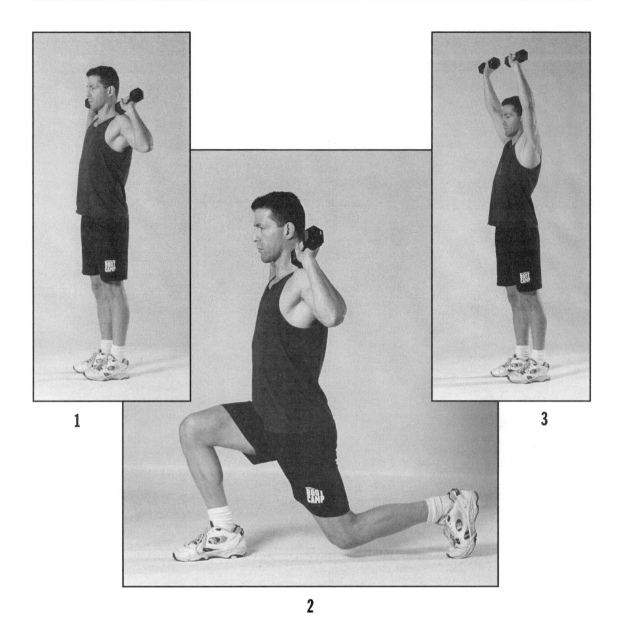

1

2

3

OVERHEAD LUNGE

Stand with your feet together, knees slightly bent. Hold two dumb bells at your shoulders. Lunge, by taking a large step in front of you with your right leg, bending it to about 90 degrees while at the same time bending your left leg so that it almost touches the floor. As you straighten out of the lunge, press both of your arms up above your head. Then return the weights to your shoulders. Repeat 15-20 times alternating your lead leg. Or do 10 times on one leg before switching to the other.

Related Daily Movement: Pushing something overhead when standing; putting heavy objects into a shelf.

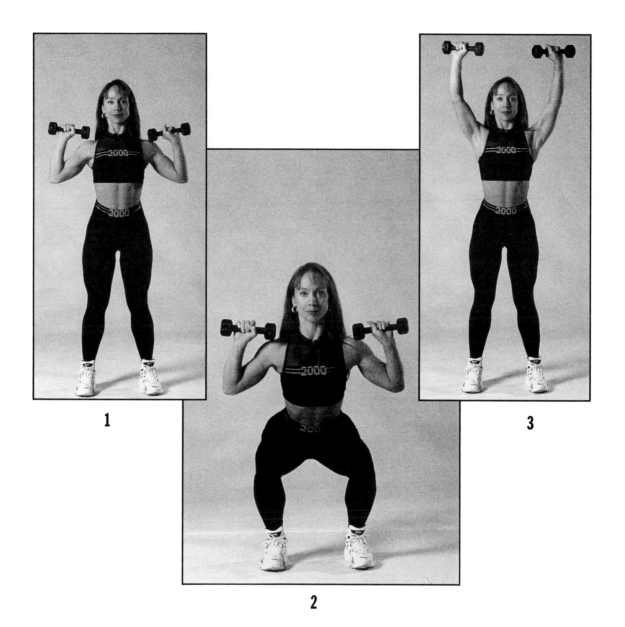

1

2

3

OVERHEAD PRESS WITH SQUAT

This exercise is the same as the overhead lunge, only instead of lunging with the weights at your shoulders, you do a squat and as you come up out of the squat press your arms up overhead. Repeat 15 times.

Related Daily Movement: Pushing something overhead when standing.

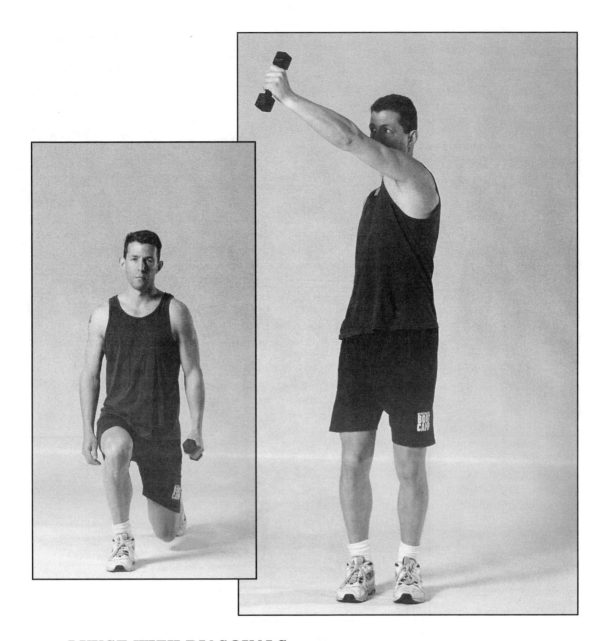

LUNGE WITH DIAGONALS

Get into a lunge, with your right leg in front of you. Hold a dumbbell down by your left leg. As you come up from the lunge, make a diagonal line with the dumbbell so that it goes above your right shoulder. Follow the dumbbell with your eyes and concentrate on using the middle or core of your body to move. Switch sides and repeat. Do 10 times on each side.

Related Daily Movements: moving in different planes, reaching across the body. Use light weights only.

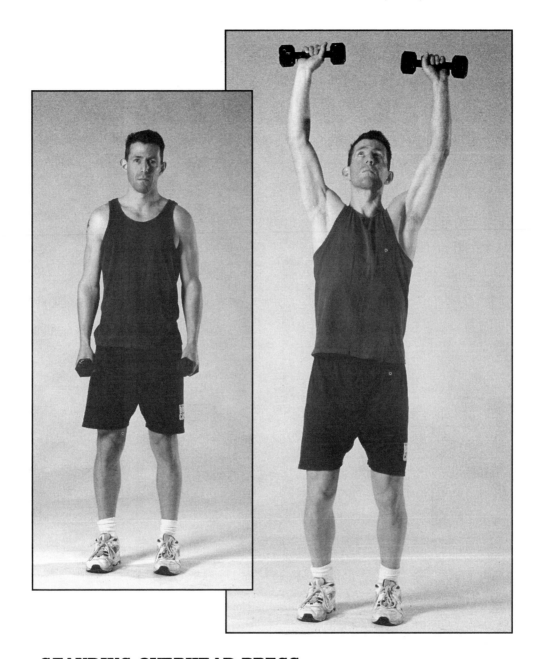

STANDING OVERHEAD PRESS

Stand with a weight in each hand. Exhale and lift the weights over head, looking up as you do so. Repeat 10-15 times.

Related Daily Movements: reaching overhead.

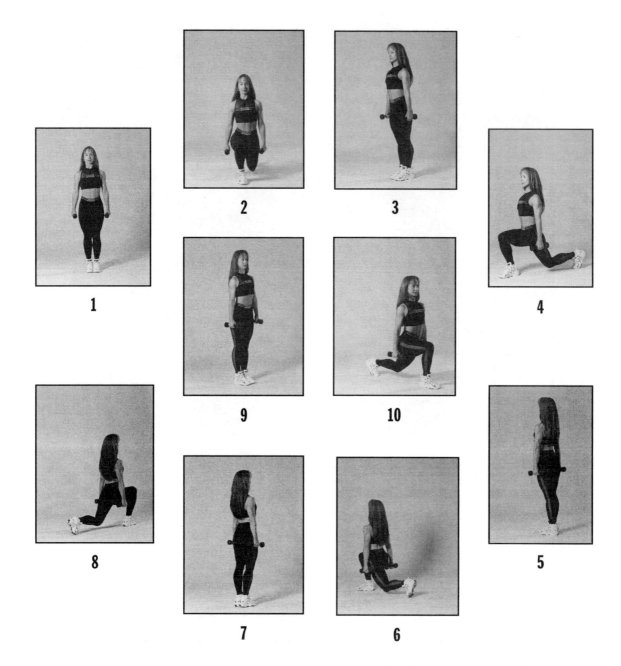

1

2

3

4

9

10

8

7

6

5

"STAR" LUNGE

Do several lunges, each at a different angle. Stand and imagine that you are in the center of a star shape. Step into a lunge so that you go into all the points of the star.

Related Daily Movements: Mobility—helping joints react to different angles.

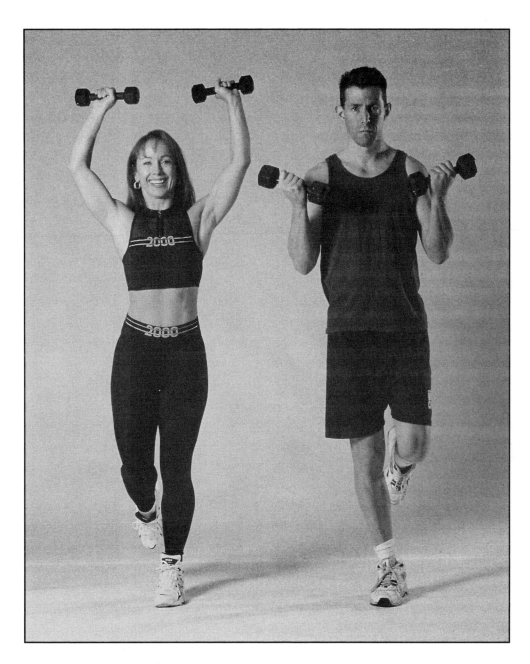

SINGLE LEG STAND

Stand on one leg while you do a traditional upper body exercise such as biceps curls or an overhead press. This is a great way to help your body stabilize from the ankles all the way up your body.

Related Daily Movement: Mobility—Balance and stability.

Warning: First try the single leg stand without using any extra weights to make sure you can balance on your own.

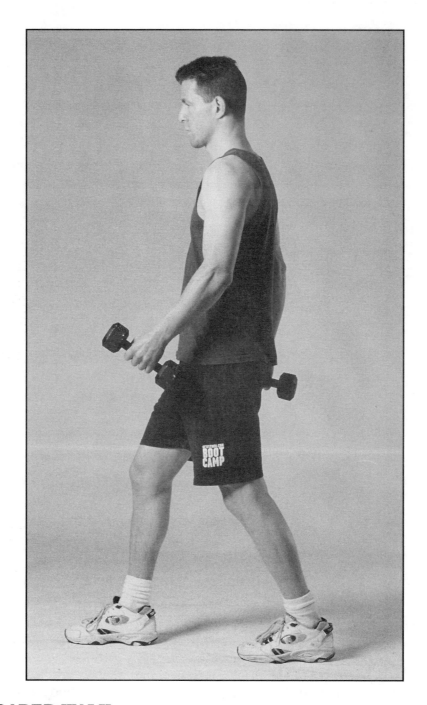

LOADED WALK

Hold weights in each hand and walk or lunge with them.

Related Daily Movements: Carrying.

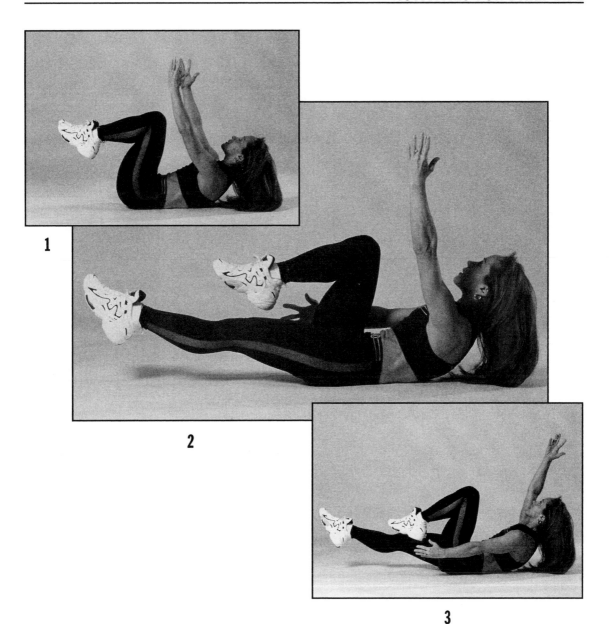

1

2

3

CORE EXERCISE

Lie on your back, maintaining your lower back's natural curve. Put both feet in the air and bend your knees. Then, put both arms straight up into the air. This is called the "dead bug" position. Nice huh? Simultaneously extend one arm and your opposite leg without losing the natural curve in your lower back. This exercise works all the muscles of the core, as opposed to only the outer abdominals. To alter the level of difficulty of this exercise you can move your arm and/or leg in varying directions.

Related Daily Movements: Virtually all, as we use our core muscles to bring about any movement.

FUNCTIONAL VS. NON FUNCTIONAL

Here are some examples of functional and non-functional exercises. As Annette Lang says, "when you are moving your own body through space" you're working out functionally. Notice how the non-functional exercises involve using a machine or being in a seated position.

FUNCTIONAL	NON-FUNCTIONAL
Squat	Hamstring Curl Machine
Lunge	Leg Extension Machine
Push-up	Bench Press
Pull-up	Seated Row
Dip	Seated Triceps Extension

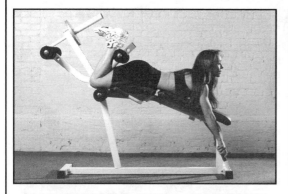

HAMSTRING CURL MACHINE

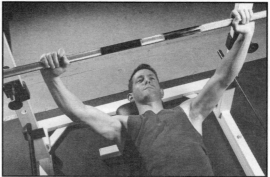

BENCH PRESS

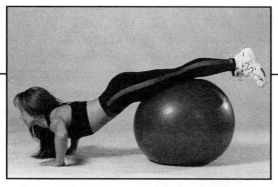

PUSH-UP ON STABILITY BALL

"I have been training with Annette for over a year and I LOVE IT! Functional training has helped me to understand more about my body and how best to use it. I used to get lower back pain, but Annette taught me how to bend down and lift things. I learned how important it is to keep my abdominals tight, and my shoulders pulled back and down. I feel that my posture has improved and I now carry myself with confidence.

Working out, while not easy, is fun. There is always something new to do that is challenging. The better I get the more I strive for perfection. It has become a priority in my life!"
—Susan P., 65 years old

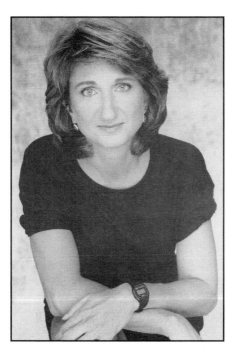

ANNETTE'S FINAL WORD:

"Remember the saying, 'It's just like riding a bike. Once you learn you never forget.' When we set up messages between the brain and the muscles through our nervous system we can remember the movements we do. Things like pull-ups, push-ups, agility drills and fun types of exercises get us back in tune with the way our body really learns to move. So have fun; relate to real life; move!"

Annette Lang, MA
Personal Trainer
National Program Director,
Esquerre Fitness Group
Educator, Reebok University

CHAPTER 6

FUNCTIONAL STRENGTH TRAINING

Traditionally, if you wanted to gain strength that meant building muscle, which also meant working out the way that bodybuilders do in the gym—isolating muscles with heavy weights through the use of machines.

By now, you realize that this is not what functional training is all about. Does this mean that if you opt for functional training you won't get the many proven benefits of aggressive strength training: a faster resting metabolism, a leaner body and muscular definition? Not at all. While the full-body focus of functional training may differ from the isolation of weight lifting, there are many exercises that you can do that are functional as well as provide enough overload or stress to your muscles to cause them to get stronger and more defined. Of course, if your ultimate goal is to be a competitive bodybuilder you will need to work out in the traditional bodybuilding way—but that's another book.

Assuming that you want to build muscle and body strength without attempting to power lift double your body weight, there is much you can do and still be working the body/brain connection that is so integral to functional training.

One note here to older exercisers: research has shown that of all types of exercising strength training is the most important to combat the gravitational effects of aging, to prevent falls and to increase functional ability. Strength gains and functional capacity have been achieved by men and women in their 80s and 90s who engage in free weight training programs.[1,2] In addition, the best programs to improve reaction times to a fall appear to be functional ones that improve power, which simply is improving speed and strength, and working on coordination.[3] So, as in the activities for daily life chapter, strength training exercises are important for you to do *whatever your age, whatever your current level of fitness.* If you are over age 30 it is important to obtain a physical before starting any exercise program and to make sure that the exercises you do are in accordance with your doctor's recommendations.

Remember that because functional training is very much tailored to the individual (not a one size fits all type of exercise), it is impossible to lay out a "standard" weight training regimen that will be effective for everyone. But there are some guidelines that can help you to create your own workout, so that the next time you go to the gym you can try to do a routine that will build strength and function at the same time. Some tips:

1. **Use free weights instead of machines whenever possible.** As discussed earlier, the reason for this is that when you use free weights many muscles of your body have to work to execute a movement. Take the biceps curl exercise as an example. If you sit at a preacher curl machine to do the biceps curl, your lower back and stomach are supported by the machine and you are only working your arms. Do the same biceps curl standing up with a free weight in each hand and you've got your abdominals and lower back muscles working to stabilize and balance your body, as well as your legs working to support you.

2. **Incorporate exercises that use medicine balls, stability balls, balance boards and other types of equipment** that help to challenge your sense of balance and develop proprioceptive awareness.

3. **Twist, bend forward and back, side to side** so that you are doing exercises in many planes.

4. If you do want to gain significant muscle mass, you may want to d**o your functional strength program two to three times a week** and then do a more traditional isolation type weight lifting program that hits all your major muscles one day a week.

5. **Great functional strength exercises include** squats, lunges, pushups, pull-ups, chin-ups, dips, standing shoulder exercises, upper body exercises using the cable crossover, standing exercises for the biceps and triceps, and of course exercises specifically that train your core muscles or that train the core in addition to other muscle groups.

6. **You only need to do one set of about 15 repetitions of each exercise.**

Christine (CC) Cunningham, owner of PerformEnhance in Chicago, has a diverse client base that ranges from athletes in their teens or 20s to men and women well over 80. She individualizes each workout based upon her clients' needs, health, goals and baseline fitness levels. CC is big on using the concepts of motor learning and control when designing an exercise program. She believes that there is a lot of confusion about functional training right now—that it has become faddish—but that once people really understand how the central nervous system works, we will see better, more effective exercise programs that will enable all of us to reach our fitness goals more efficiently.

"When someone is learning a movement, there are things that happen on both subconscious and conscious levels," CC explains. "For example, if a person is learning how to do a bench press (lying on a bench, you press weight up above your chest), initially his brain is trying to figure out which muscles to use and when—just to make the lift look right. During this phase of the learning process, you can only ask him to attend to one thing at a time, such as making sure that his back doesn't rise up. If you try to make it too complicated, he won't learn it properly."

This is important, because we learn by mastering one thing at a time. In the functional training craze, CC has seen people rush to perform more complicated and involved exercises, such as lunging while pressing weights overhead. This can lead to injury. "It is important to attend to one skill until it becomes automatic and then move on to incorporating other things," she warns. Otherwise, there is an increased risk of injury in addition to a decrease in effectiveness.

Because of the stepped way in which we learn, CC often uses basic lifting first, so that proper breathing and basic movement patterns become automatic. In addition, she is careful not to cue her clients too much, because the brain will actually become dependent on a trainer's cue in order to perform a movement. This is fine when you're actually in the training session, but may prevent you from taking what you learn in the gym and using it in real life which, of course, is the ultimate goal of functional training.

CC also sees value in doing isolation exercises with some of her clients and argues that there definitely are times when they would be considered functional, even though they only involve one muscle group. "Say your left biceps is weaker than your right biceps and you insist on doing a pull-up because it's considered more 'functional' than an isolated biceps curl. Well, your brain will send messages to use the right biceps (the stronger muscle) more and you'll never gain strength in the left biceps to even the two out. So, in a case like that I would recommend doing isolation work for the left biceps, until it gains strength," she explains.

CC CUNNINGHAM'S FUNCTIONAL STRENGTH TRAINING WORKOUT

CC has designed a sample program that you may use as a guide. She has created this program for a woman in her early 30s, with two toddlers, who wants to increase her tone and improve her ability to do her everyday activities associated with caring for her children (primarily lifting and carrying).

THE PROGRAM

Times Per Week: One to two days per week, supplementing with one additional time per week doing a traditional machine weight training program.

Amount of Weight: Moderate, based on weakest point in range of motion or on body weight.

Repetitions: 12-20 of each exercise or until proper form breaks down.

Sets: One.

Speed: Quick controlled acceleration (as you would in life) with full range of motion.

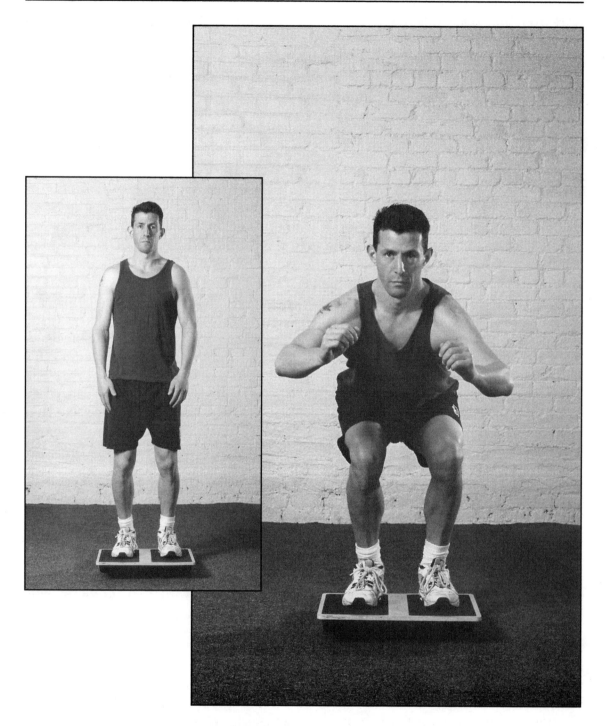

BALANCE BOARD SQUATS

Perform a squat while standing on a balance board. To challenge yourself even more, do the same exercise while you hold a medicine ball in various positions.

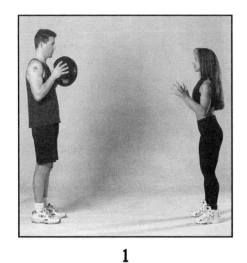

1

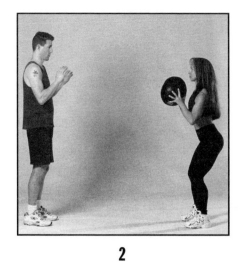

2

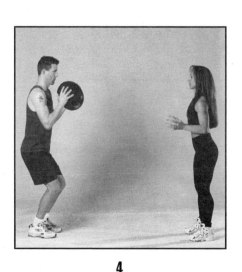

3

4

MEDICINE BALL CHEST PRESS

Stand with your knees bent slightly over your toes, toss a medicine ball to a partner and then have the partner toss it back to you. Make sure you initiate the toss from your legs.

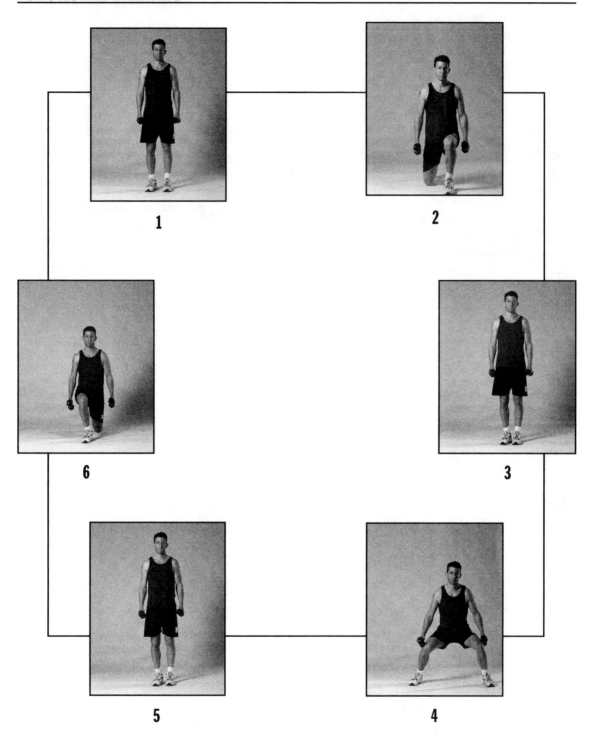

MULTI DIRECTIONAL LUNGES

Lunge with one leg in at least three directions, forward, out to the side and behind you (you may also lunge to all positions in-between these). Switch to the other leg.

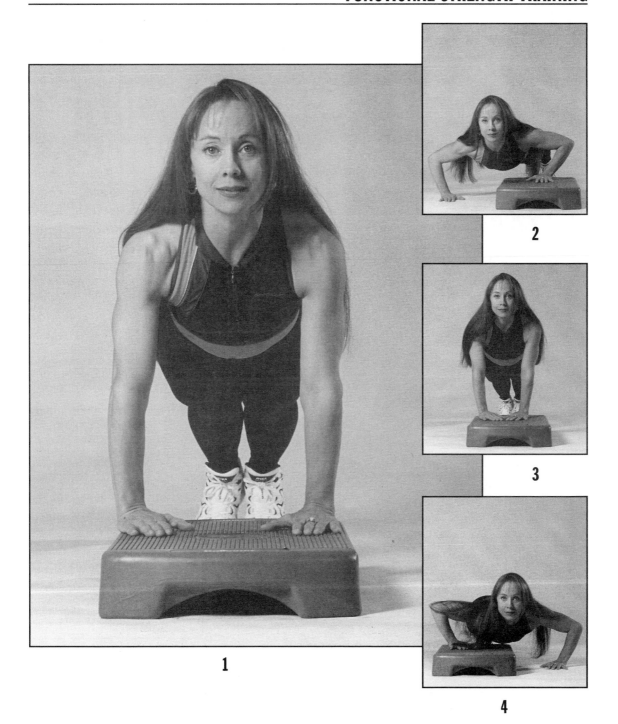

1

2

3

4

STEP OUT PUSH-UP

Place both hands on a raised platform or bench, move both your right hand and right leg out to the side simultaneously. Then, focus on lowering your chest in a controlled manner and quickly pushing back up to the original position. Repeat, this time moving your left hand and left leg.

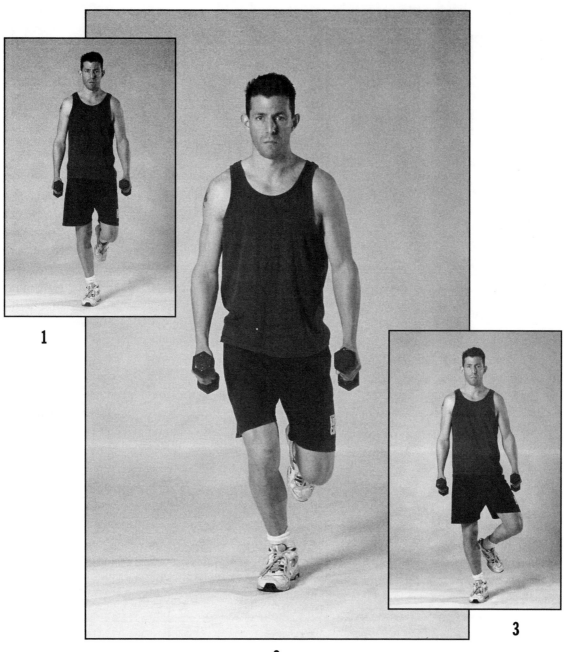

1

2

3

SINGLE LEG HALF SQUATS
Stand on one leg and perform a squat (only go halfway down). Repeat, changing the position of your bent leg to work more on balance and stabilization.

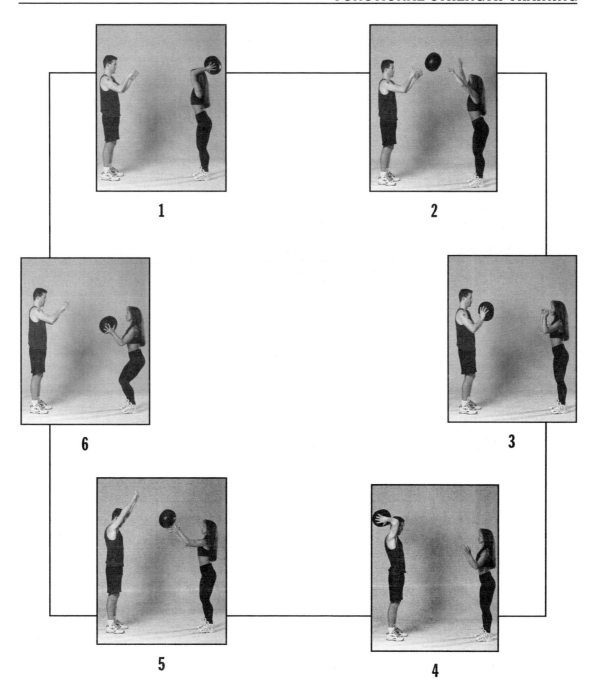

1 2

6 3

5 4

MEDICINE BALL OVERHEAD TOSS

Stand with your hips square and knees slightly bent. Initiating movement from your legs, and being careful not to keep your abdominals pulled in tight, toss a medicine ball over your head to a partner's chest; catch the ball.

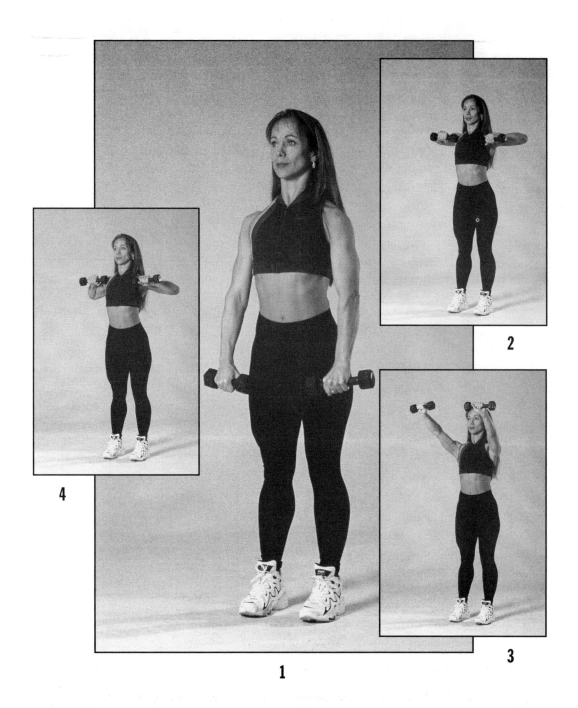

1

2

3

4

DIAGONAL ROW

Stand, holding a dumbbell in each hand; lift your hands to your chest, performing an upright row. Then, push your arms out to a 45-degree overhead press. Focus on stabilizing your torso, and moving in a fluid, controlled manner. Return and repeat.

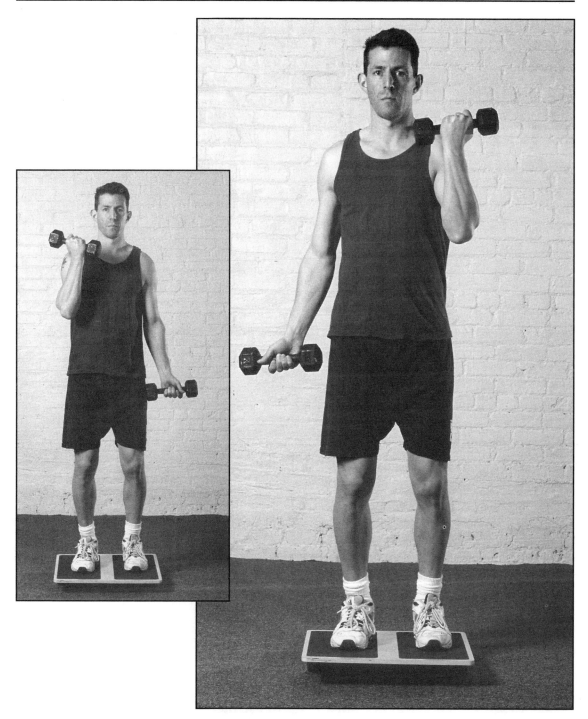

BICEPS ON THE BOARD

Stand on a balance board and perform alternating biceps curls, focusing on keeping your torso stabilized, and balance. Do some exercises with your shoulders turned in, then do some with your shoulders rotated outward.

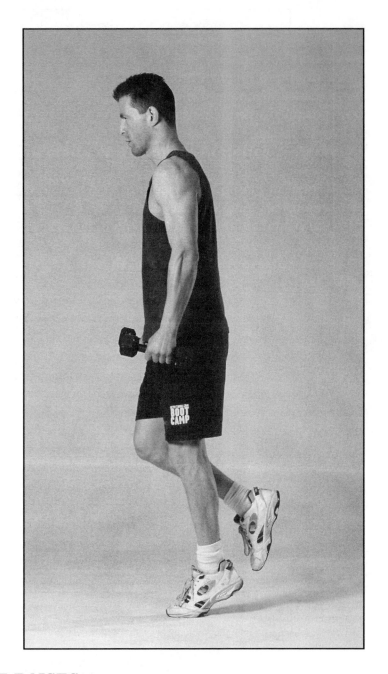

CALF RAISES

Balance on one leg. Lift quickly up to the ball of your foot and concentrate on balancing. Lower and repeat. Switch to other leg.

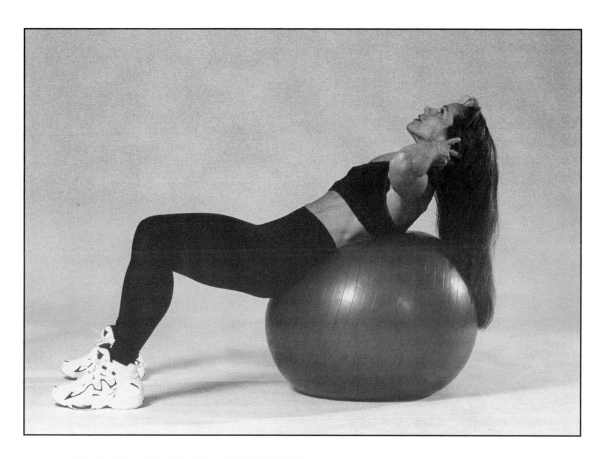

STABILITY BALL CRUNCHES

Sit on a stability ball, move your body down until your lower back is on the ball. From this position, with your arms crossed in front of your chest or behind your head, lift your torso performing a crunch. Then lower back to slight stretch of the abdomen.

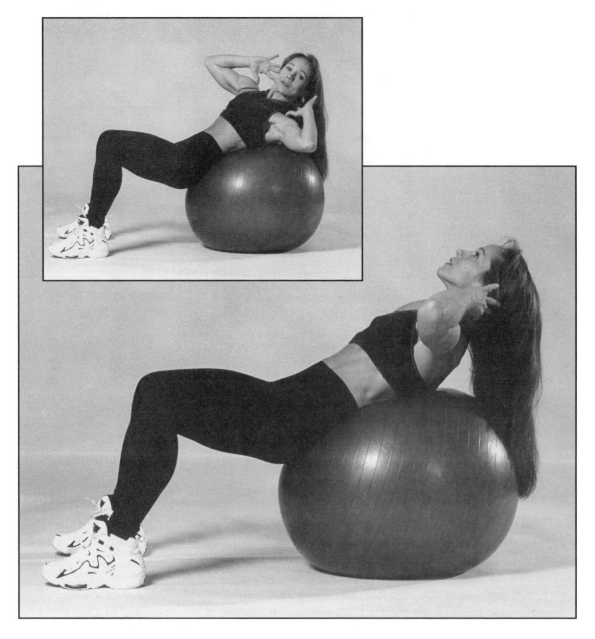

STABILITY BALL OBLIQUES

Perform a crunch from on top of a stability ball, this time adding a twist to each side.

IN A FUNCTIONAL EXERCISE YOUR BODY MOVES (ACCELERATES, DECELERATES OR STABILIZES) IN THESE THREE PLANES:

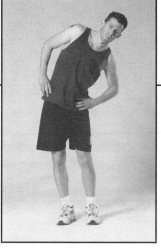

FRONTAL PLANE
bending at the waist
from side to side

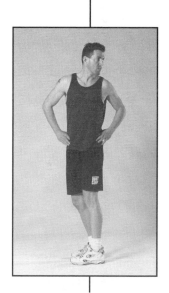

TRANSVERSE PLANE
twisting your body

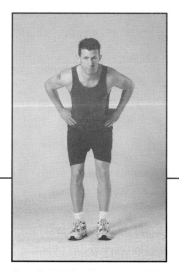

SAGGITAL PLANE
bending your body
forward and
backwards

"I've been training with CC for over a year now. I'm a mountain bike racer and want to get into cycle cross racing, which is a one mile closed-loop bike race that involves obstacles. It's very, very challenging. Bike racing requires power, balance and control, so CC and I work a lot on balance, agility, coordination and power moves. For power I started running and doing plyometrics. We do dynamic strength training: foot work drills, goose kicks, things like that.

I wish that I knew about functional training when I was an athlete in school. All we did then was run, practice and lift weights. I am so much more fit now. I recently went biking in Canada and noticed how much better I can climb. I see a huge difference in my performance now!"

—Lisa Bourazak, mountain bike racer, Chicago, IL.

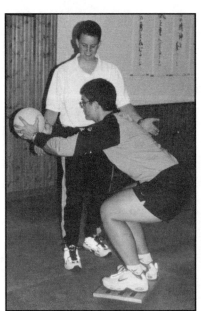

CC'S FINAL WORD:

"When determining a functional exercise, consider the risks versus the benefits. If you notice your body doesn't feel so good after a workout, reconsider what you're doing. Functional training can be risky, especially if you're doing dynamic movements with weights. I'm a big advocate of 'if it feels good, go with it.'"

Christine (CC) Cunningham, MS, ATC/L
Owner PerformEnhance
Evanston, IL
Telephone: 847-733-0962
E-mail: ccunningham@performenhance.net
Website: performenhance.net

CHAPTER 7

PROGRAMS FOR ATHLETES

"We never realized we were doing functional training. It was just part of our overall training program with athletes."
      —Vern Gambetta, director of Gambetta Sports Training Systems.

You're an athlete. There is a particular sport in which you participate on a regular basis, perhaps even on a competitive basis. To say that you "play" that sport would be a gross understatement—you're so passionate about it—you practically eat, drink and breathe it. In fact, you never feel better than when you're volleying on a tennis court, skiing downhill or running across a field.

Of course, as a dedicated athlete you're always looking to improve your performance on the court, slopes or field. You may have tried going to the gym, lifting heavier and heavier weights, but find that your newly acquired behemoth biceps are doing squat for your game. Likewise, you may find that all the step aerobics and spinning that you thought were going to make you impenetrable on the field haven't much changed the way you play. While these other activities may be great cross training and may help to improve your overall fitness levels, to improve your performance in your sport of preference you need to train in a way that is functional.

Remember, since the athletic training we are discussing in this chapter is a type of functional training, the activity must be specific to the actual event, so it is not possible to create a single program that will improve performance for all athletes in all sports. However, we can generally recognize that athletes will benefit by incorporating agility training, speed training, coordination training and a vertical jump improvement program into their training. The specifics involved in each program will need to vary depending upon several factors, including your level of ability, your goals, and the actual sport for which you are training.

One general way in which you can improve your agility, speed, coordination and jumping ability is by doing boot camp style sports conditioning workouts. Generally given in a group exercise format, but also possible to do one-on-one with a trainer, boot camp workouts are intense and energetic, and are modeled after military workout regimens. Sessions include intervals of plyometric training (which improves your ability to perform powerful jumps), speed and coordination drills, and functional strength training through exercises such as push-ups, bench dips, squats and lunges. If you want to improve your overall athletic skill set, ask your trainer to use this type of training with you, or check out a sports conditioning/boot camp class.

When it comes to coaching athletes to get them to achieve their best performance, you'd be hard pressed to find someone with better credentials than Vern Gambetta. Vern has served as speed and conditioning coach for the Tampa Bay Mutiny Major League Soccer Team, conditioning consultant to the U.S. Men's World Cup Team and the New England Revolution, as well as director of conditioning for the Chicago White Sox. His experience and success as a coach and fitness professional over more than 31 years have gained him international recognition as an expert in training and conditioning for sports, and he is sought after worldwide as a fitness speaker and lecturer. In this chapter, Vern shares some of his great body of knowledge in the area of functional sports training and conditioning to help you realize your performance potential as an athlete.

As Vern says in the preface to this book, "the body is a link system," meaning that in order to truly do exercise that is functional, we must concentrate not on individual muscles, but on how those muscles work together to create movement. Movement occurs in three planes, the saggital (bending forward and back, or flexion/extension), the frontal (bending side to side) and the transverse (rotation or twisting). Sports require movement in all three planes. While it would make sense then that athletic training should involve multi-plane movement, traditionally this has not been the case.

"We were all educated that rotation was bad," explains Vern. "Yet, if you analyze life skills and sports, rotation is key. We must work in all three planes. Initially I did a lot of isolation work with athletes and found that they weren't doing as well as they should," he says. "I started looking into physical therapy and my eyes were opened to less isolation and more integrated movement." He began to incorporate multi-plane, multi-joint training that was high in proprioceptive demand (challenging to the receptors that we have in our tendons and joints) and started to see amazing improvements in his athletes.

"To determine the types of functional exercise you should do is extremely individualistic, it depends upon your sports goal and is directly related to the type of stress you place your body under everyday in your sport," he explains. Vern suggests that you ask yourself about the following issues to determine what you should do:

- The demands of your sport (does it require jumping ability, speed, endurance?)

- What position you are in now and where you want to be.

- Look at the qualities you have and where you need to improve.

- Determine the typical injury patterns of your sport and develop an exer
cise that addresses these areas. (For example, if you are a tennis player
and are at risk for elbow strain you want to make sure that your program
involves exercises to strengthen your arms.)

As Vern says, "functional training is not a shot in the dark. It is not one size
fits all." You should consider the issues above and then work with a fitness professional to develop a routine that will help you to meet your goals. However,
since jumping is a key skill that athletes in a myriad of sports need to master,
Vern provides the following vertical jump improvement program for you.

VERN GAMBETTA'S
VERTICAL JUMP IMPROVEMENT PROGRAM

"The main stimulus to improve jumping power is intensity. The following
detailed program I developed is characterized by relatively low volume (the total
number of repetitions) in all the plyometric exercises as well as a small menu of
supplementary exercises in strength training and speed training. The strength
training and speed training are supplementary to the jumping exercises
because the focus of this particular program is to improve your vertical jumping
ability. The supplementary activities are designed to stimulate your nervous
system.

"Plyometric training is not meant as a conditioning activity. Its main goal is
to improve explosive power. In order to accomplish that goal the emphasis must
be on the quality of movement and explosiveness. Another key to improving
your jump is to eliminate aerobic work because it dulls the nervous system. In
essence, if you do plyometric work and aerobic work during the same session,
you are creating confusion in your brain."

This program is very simple. First you will find a visual description of some
major exercises. At the end of the chapter is Vern Gambetta's six-week progres-
sive program. "Consistency is the key. Execute each movement with precision.
Aim for explosiveness and speed of movement on each repetition." Enjoy!

EXERCISES

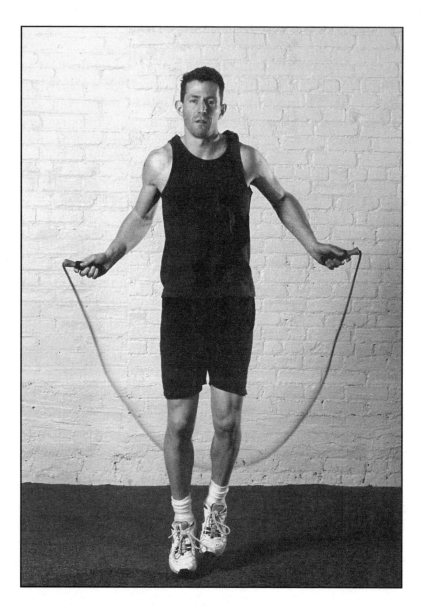

JUMP ROPE
Perform a controlled series of jumps.

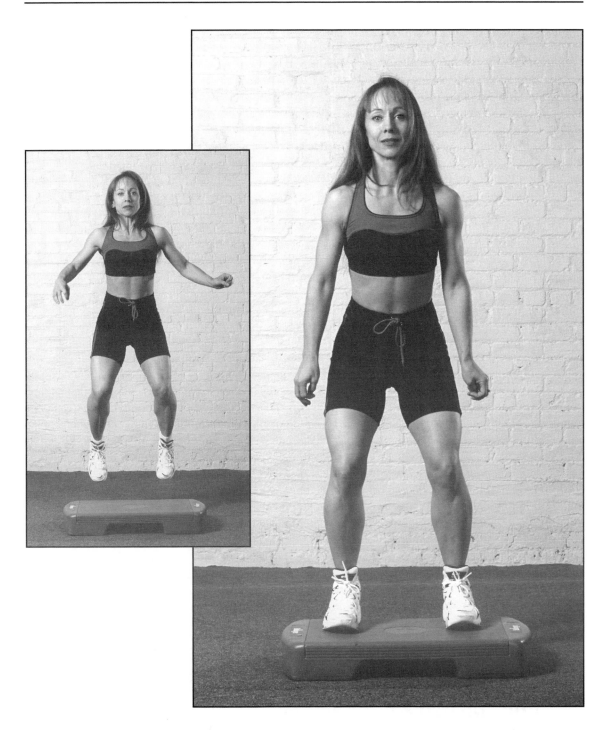

JUMP AND STICK
Jump up onto a platform; make sure you land on both feet.

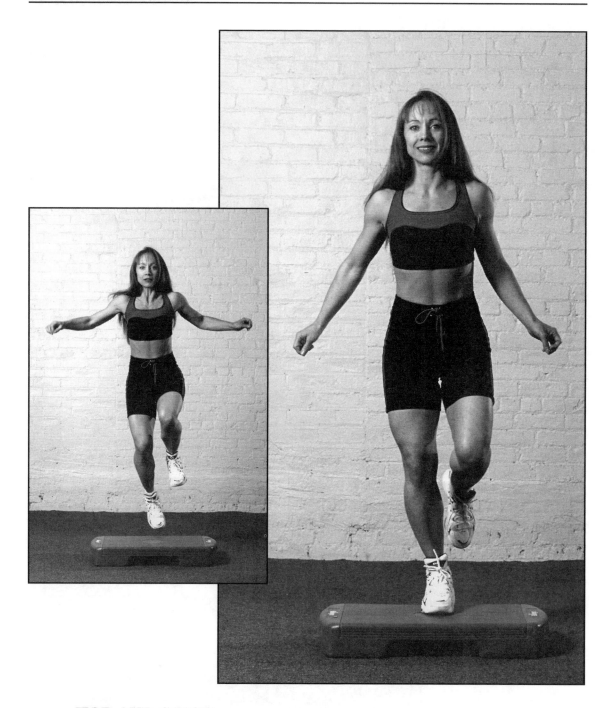

HOP AND STICK

Jump up onto a platform, landing on one leg. Hold your hands out for balance.

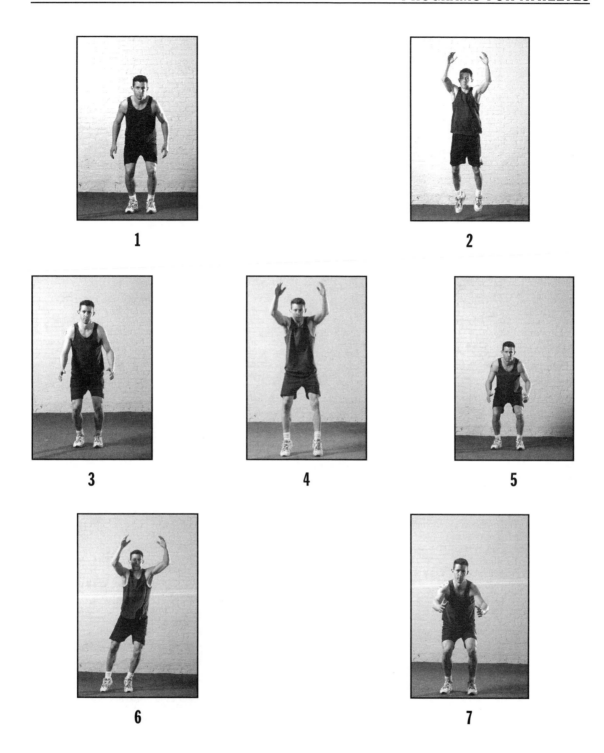

MULTI DIRECTIONAL JUMPS
Jump in several directions.

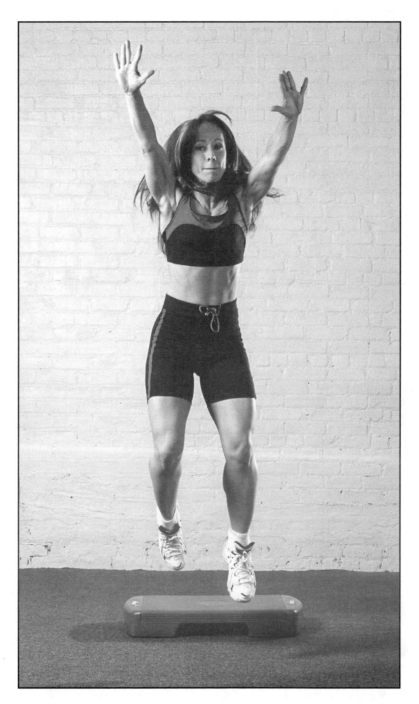

VERTICAL JUMP
Step off a bench onto the floor, then jump up as high as you can.

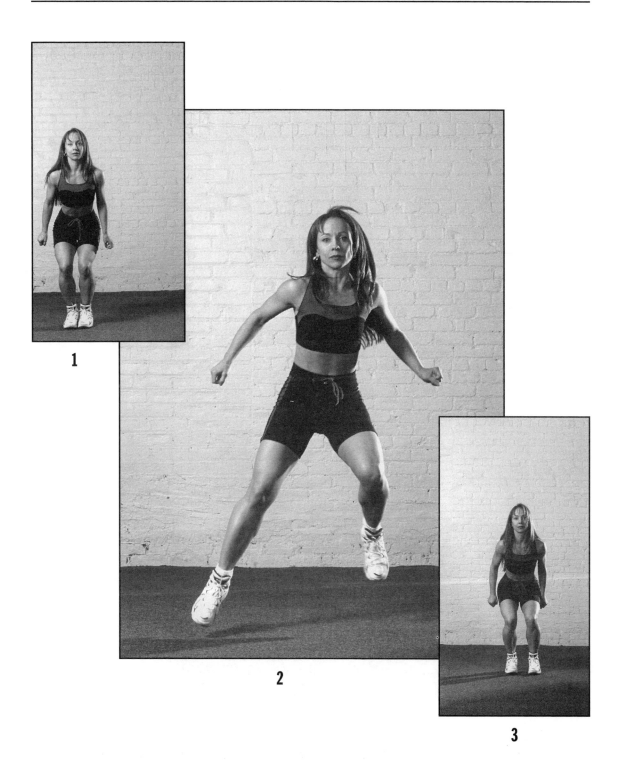

1

2

3

STEP CLOSE

Step with one leg out to the side; jump to bring the other leg in.

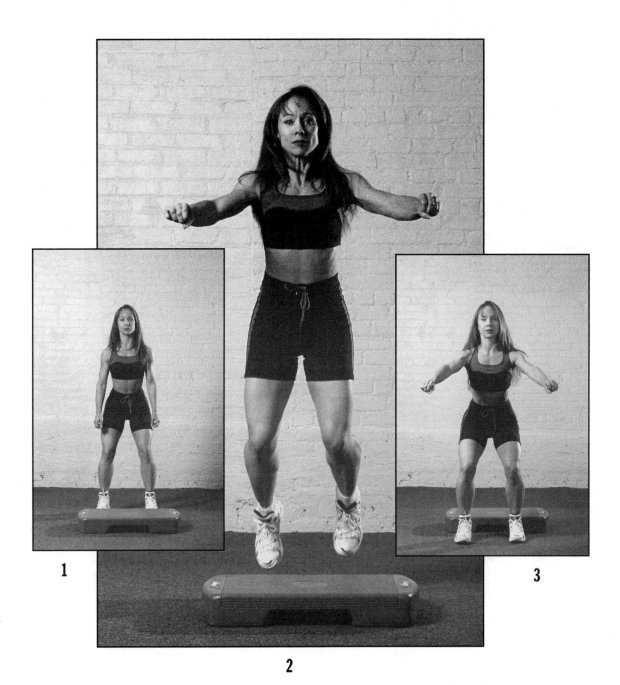

1

2

3

HURDLE JUMP
Squat behind a box or bench, then execute a jump over the hurdle.

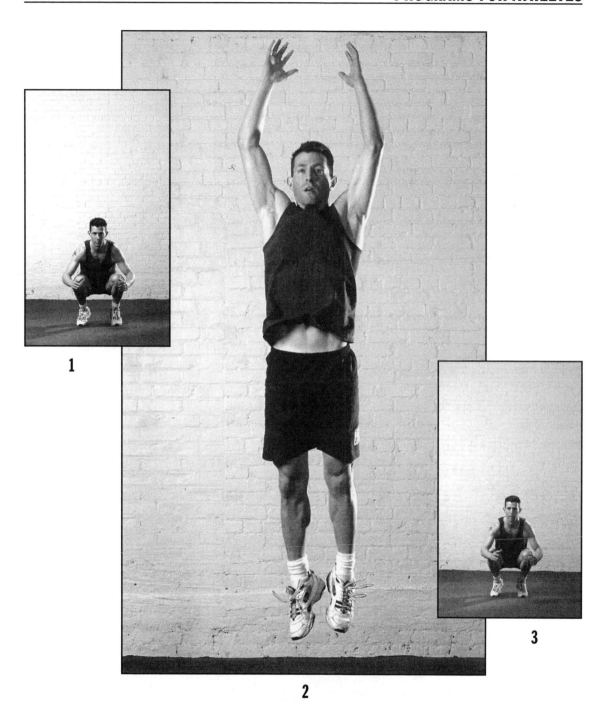

1

2

3

SQUAT JUMP

Assume a squat position; jump as high as you can before returning to the squat.

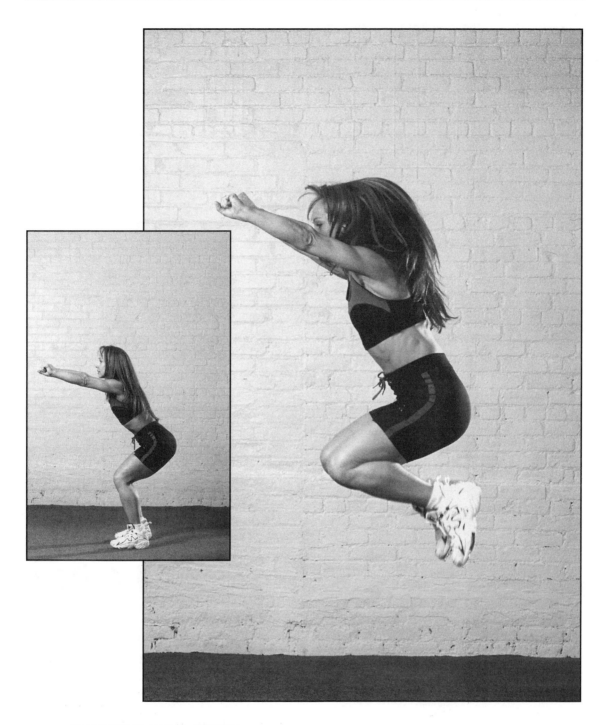

DOUBLE LEG JUMP

From squat position, jump up, bringing your heels into your butt.

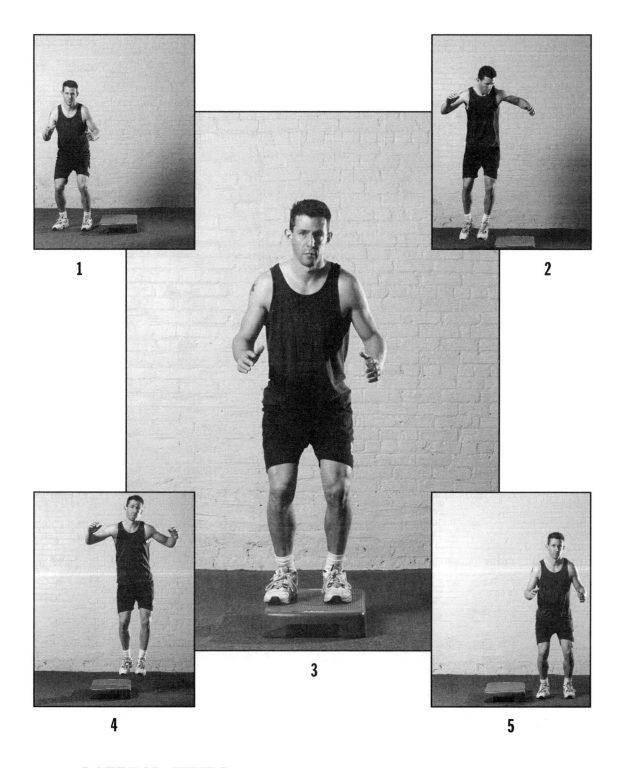

1

2

3

4

5

LATERAL JUMPS

Stand at one side of bench, jump up, then quickly jump off to the other side.

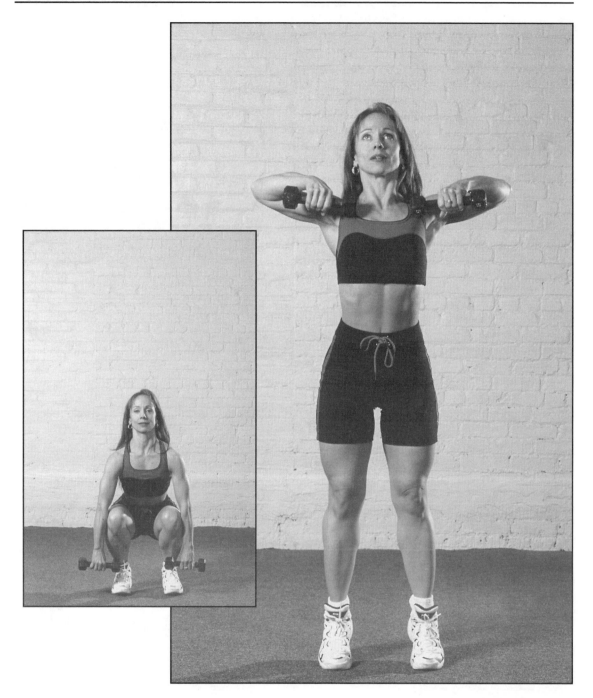

DUMBBELL HIGH PULL

Begin in squat position with dumbbells in your hands; as you straighten your legs, bend your arms, bringing your hands to your chest.

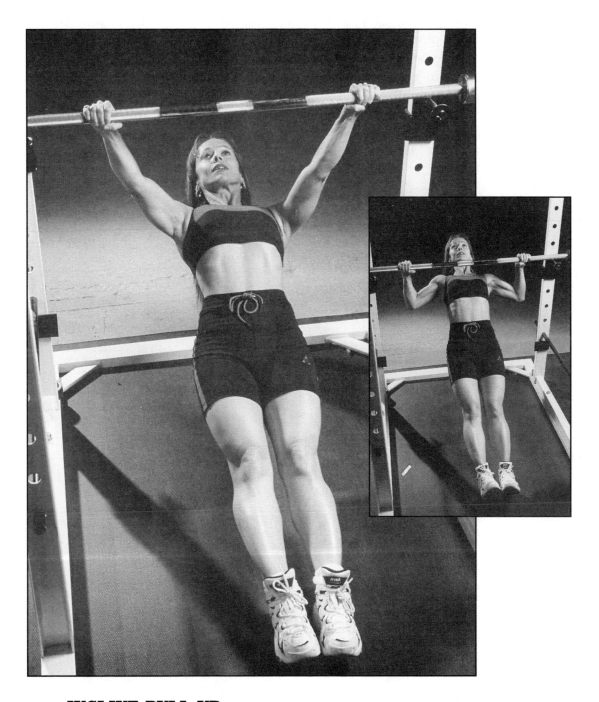

INCLINE PULL-UP

Perform a modified pull-up by positioning yourself under the bar. Hold the bar using either the regular or reverse grip. Straighten your back, hips, and legs and pull your chest to the bar.

Vern believes that while people are looking at high levels of athletic performance as the model that they ultimately want to embrace, they need to consider their own unique situations. He notes that the basic reality of gravity is the same for world-class athlete, weekend warrior or sedentary person. As we age, gravity begins to get an advantage that can be significantly kept in check through functional strength training.

"If you are older it is far more important to do strength training and flexibility training. If you are a woman you need to do more strength training at a younger age and do it often to prevent osteoporosis," advises Vern.

Just as it makes no sense to get on a direct flight to Los Angeles if your desired destination is Chicago, it makes no sense to do high speed drills if you're deconditioned and really in need of functional strength. The bottom line: assess where you are, determine where you want or need to be, and do the appropriate functional training to get you there!

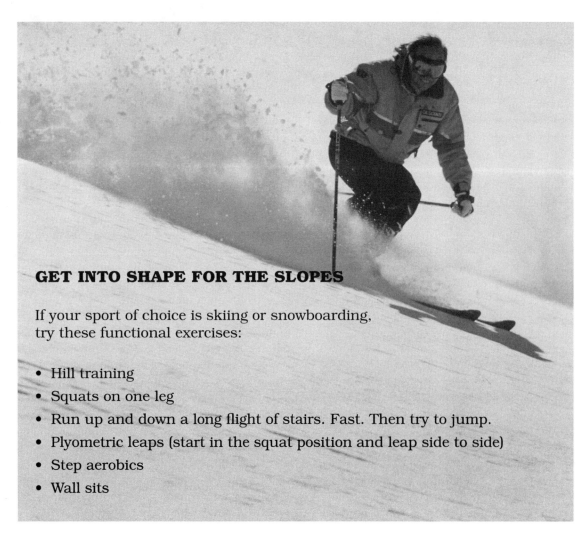

GET INTO SHAPE FOR THE SLOPES

If your sport of choice is skiing or snowboarding,
try these functional exercises:

- Hill training
- Squats on one leg
- Run up and down a long flight of stairs. Fast. Then try to jump.
- Plyometric leaps (start in the squat position and leap side to side)
- Step aerobics
- Wall sits

PHOTO CREDIT: FROM ANYONE CAN BE AN

"Vern Gambetta has made me a better coach. He has the courage and intelligence to constantly submit conventional wisdom and training trends to the acid test of absolute performance. Beyond that, he is a true coach: somebody with real knowledge and experience, and an eagerness and ability to share them."

—Steve Myrland, coach, University of Wisconsin Athletics

"Vern Gambetta has been an immense help to myself and others in helping sort out the necessary from the 'nice to do' in functional training. He takes both an academic and practical application approach to the subject which is well grounded."

—Gary Winckler, women's track and field coach, University of Illinois

VERN'S FINAL WORD:

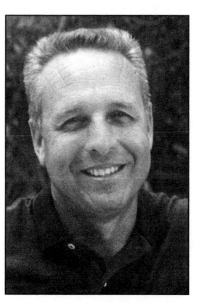

"Functional training is not doing crazy things with new tools. Just because you are using a stability ball does not mean that you necessarily are doing a functional exercise. For example, doing squats on a stability ball is not so functional. You're better off doing squats on the floor.

"In my view functional training is the only way to go. For weight loss you can do activities that are as active and involve as much movement as possible. Keep in mind that functional training has a higher caloric expenditure than isolation training. For everyday life activities functional training helps combat low back pain, carpal tunnel syndrome and neck pain; as for athletic performance: it is necessary beyond question!"

Vern Gambetta, MA
Gambetta Sports Training Systems
Website: gambetta.com
Telephone: 800-671-4045

VERN GAMBETTA'S SIX-WEEK TRAINING PROGRAM

WEEK #1

DAY 1

Jump Training

Jump Rope	3 x	25
Jump & Stick	1 x	10
Hop & Stick	2 x	10
Multidirectional	2 x	8
Jump Ups	2 x	10
Vertical Jump	3 x	5
Step Close	3 x	5
Hurdle Jump 24"	5 x	5
Squat Jump	3 x	12

Weight Training

Push-up	2 x	5
DB High Pull	3 x	6
DB Bench Press	3 x	8
Incline Pull-up	3 x	10
Pull-down	3 x	8
Leg Circuit	2 x	1

Speed Training

10 yrd Sprint	1 x	10
5-10-5	1 x	5
Speed Ladder	5 x	1

DAY 2

Jump Training

Jump Rope	4 x	25
Jump & Stick	1 x	10
Hop & Stick	2 x	10
Multidirectional	2 x	8
Jump Ups	3 x	10
Vertical Jump	3 x	5
Step Close	3 x	5
Double Leg Jump	3 x	5
Band Jump	3 x	10

Weight Training

Push-up	2 x	5
DB Push Press	3 x	6
Incline Pull-up	3 x	8

Speed Training

10 yrd Sprint	1 x	10
5-10-5	1 x	5
Speed Ladder	5 x	1

DAY 3

Jump Training

Jump Rope	5 x	25
Jump & Stick	1 x	10
Hop & Stick	2 x	10
Multidirectional	2 x	8
Jump Ups	4 x	10
Vertical Jump	2 x	5
Step Close	2 x	5
Band Jump	4 x	8
Squat Jump	3 x	15

Weight Training

Push-up	2 x	5
DB High Pull	3 x	6
DB Bench Press	3 x	6
Incline Pull-up	3 x	8
Pull-down	3 x	6
Leg Circuit	3 x	1

Speed Training

VERN GAMBETTA'S SIX-WEEK TRAINING PROGRAM

WEEK #2

DAY 1			
Jump Training			
Jump Rope	3	x	25
Jump & Stick	1	x	10
Hop & Stick	2	x	10
Multidirectional	2	x	8
Vertical Jump	3	x	5
Step Close	3	x	5
Hurdle Jump 24"	5	x	5
Squat Jump	3	x	18
Weight Training			
Push-up	2	x	5
DB High Pull	3	x	6
DB Bench Press	3	x	8
Incline Pull-up	3	x	10
Pull-down	3	x	8
Leg Circuit	2	x	1
Speed Training			
10 yrd Sprint	1	x	10
5-10-5	1	x	5
Speed Ladder	5	x	1

DAY 2			
Jump Training			
Jump Rope	4	x	25
Jump & Stick	1	x	10
Hop & Stick	2	x	10
Multidirectional	2	x	8
Vertical Jump	3	x	5
Step Close	3	x	5
Double Leg Jump	5	x	5
Band Jump	4	x	10
Weight Training			
Push-up	2	x	5
DB Push Press	3	x	6
Pull-down	3	x	8
Incline Pull-up	3	x	10
Speed Training			
10 yrd Sprint	1	x	10
5-10-5	1	x	5
Speed Ladder	5	x	1

DAY 3			
Jump Training			
Jump Rope	5	x	25
Jump & Stick	1	x	10
Hop & Stick	2	x	10
Multidirectional	2	x	8
Vertical Jump	2	x	5
Step Close	2	x	5
Band Jump	5	x	8
Squat Jump	3	x	15
Weight Training			
Push-up	2	x	5
DB High Pull	3	x	6
DB Bench Press	3	x	6
Incline Pull-up	3	x	10
Pull-down	3	x	6
Leg Circuit	3	x	1
Speed Training			
none			

VERN GAMBETTA'S SIX-WEEK TRAINING PROGRAM

WEEK #3

DAY 1			
Jump Training			
Jump Rope	3	x	25
Jump & Stick	1	x	10
Hop & Stick	2	x	10
Multidirectional	2	x	8
Jump Ups	3	x	5
Step Close	3	x	5
Hurdle Jump 24"	5	x	10
Squat Jump	3	x	15
Weight Training			
Push-up	2	x	5
DB High Pull	3	x	6
DB Bench Press	3	x	8
Incline Pull-up	3	x	10
Pull-down	3	x	8
Leg Circuit	2	x	1
Speed Training			
10 yrd Sprint	1	x	10
5-10-5	1	x	5
Speed Ladder	5	x	1

DAY 2			
Jump Training			
Jump Rope	4	x	25
Jump & Stick	1	x	10
Hop & Stick	2	x	10
Multidirectional	2	x	8
Jump Ups	3	x	5
Step Close	3	x	5
Double Leg Jump	5	x	5
Band Jump	5	x	10
Weight Training			
Push-up	2	x	5
DB Push Press	3	x	6
Pull-down	3	x	8
Incline Pull-up	3	x	8
Speed Training			
10 yrd Sprint	1	x	10
5-10-5	1	x	5
Speed Ladder	5	x	1

DAY 3			
Jump Training			
Jump Rope	5	x	25
Jump & Stick	1	x	10
Hop & Stick	2	x	10
Multidirectional	2	x	8
Vertical Jump	2	x	5
Step Close	2	x	5
Band Jump	5	x	8
Squat Jump	3	x	15
Weight Training			
Push-up	2	x	5
DB High Pull	3	x	6
Pull-down	3	x	6
DB Bench Press	3	x	6
Incline Pull-up	3	x	8
Leg Circuit	3	x	1
Speed Training			
none			

VERN GAMBETTA'S SIX-WEEK TRAINING PROGRAM

WEEK #4

DAY 1		

Jump Training

Jump Rope	3 x	25
Jump & Stick	1 x	10
Hop & Stick	2 x	10
Multidirectional	2 x	8
Vertical Jump	5 x	5
Step Close	3 x	5
Hurdle Jump 24"	5 x	10
Squat Jump	3 x	15

Weight Training

Push-up	3 x	5
DB High Pull	3 x	4
Squat	4 x	6
Step Up (each leg)	3 x	8
DB Bench Press	4 x	6

Speed Training

10 yrd Sprint	2 x	10
5-10-5	1 x	5
Speed Ladder	5 x	1

DAY 2		

Jump Training

Jump Rope	4 x	25
Jump & Stick	1 x	10
Hop & Stick	2 x	10
Multidirectional	2 x	8
Vertical Jump	3 x	5
Step Close	3 x	5
Double Leg Jump	5 x	5
Band Jump	3 x	10

Weight Training

Push-up	4 x	5
DB Push Press	3 x	4
Pull-down	4 x	6
Incline Pull-up	3 x	8

Speed Training

10 yrd Sprint	2 x	10
5-10-5	1 x	5
Speed Ladder	5 x	1

DAY 3		

Jump Training

Jump Rope	5 x	25
Jump & Stick	1 x	10
Hop & Stick	2 x	10
Multidirectional	2 x	8
Vertical Jump	5 x	5
Step Close	2 x	5
Band Jump	5 x	8
Squat Jump	3 x	18

Weight Training

Push-up	3 x	5
DB High Pull	4 x	4
Squat	5 x	6
Step Up (each leg)	3 x	6
DB Bench Press	3 x	6

Speed Training

VERN GAMBETTA'S SIX-WEEK TRAINING PROGRAM

WEEK #5

DAY 1		

Jump Training

Jump Rope	3 x 25
Jump & Stick	1 x 10
Hop & Stick	2 x 10
Multidirectional	2 x 8
Vertical Jump	5 x 5
Step Close	3 x 5
Hurdle Jump 28"	5 x 10
Squat Jump	3 x 21

Weight Training

Push-up	3 x 5
DB High Pull	3 x 4
Squat	4 x 6
Step Up (each leg)	3 x 8
DB Bench Press	4 x 6

Speed Training

10 yrd Sprint	1 x 10
5-10-5	1 x 5
Speed Ladder	5 x 1

DAY 2		

Jump Training

Jump Rope	4 x 25
Jump & Stick	1 x 10
Hop & Stick	2 x 10
Multidirectional	2 x 8
Vertical Jump	3 x 5
Step Close	3 x 5
Band Jump	3 x 10

Weight Training

Push-up	4 x 5
DB Push Press	3 x 4
Pull-down	4 x 6
Pull-up	3 x 8

Speed Training

10 yrd Sprint	1 x 10
5-10-5	1 x 5
Speed Ladder	5 x 1

DAY 3		

Jump Training

Jump Rope	5 x 25
Jump & Stick	1 x 10
Hop & Stick	2 x 10
Multidirectional	2 x 8
Vertical Jump	5 x 5
Hurdle Jump 28"	5 x 10
Squat Jump	3 x 24

Weight Training

Push-up	3 x 5
DB High Pull	4 x 4
Squat	5 x 6
Step Up (each leg)	3 x 6
DB Bench Press	3 x 6
Pull-down	4 x 6

Speed Training

VERN GAMBETTA'S SIX-WEEK TRAINING PROGRAM

WEEK #6

DAY 1

Jump Training

Jump Rope	3	x	25
Jump & Stick	1	x	10
Hop & Stick	2	x	10
Multidirectional	2	x	8
Vertical Jump	5	x	3
Step Close	3	x	3
Hurdle Jump 28"	3	x	10
Squat Jump	3	x	27

Weight Training

Push-up	3	x	5
DB High Pull	3	x	4
Squat	4	x	6
Step Up (each leg)	3	x	8
DB Bench Press	4	x	6

Speed Training

10 yrd Sprint	1	x	10
5-10-5	1	x	5
Speed Ladder	5	x	1

DAY 2

Jump Training

Jump Rope	4	x	25
Jump & Stick	1	x	10
Hop & Stick	2	x	10
Multidirectional	2	x	8
Vertical Jump	3	x	5
Step Close	3	x	5
Band Jump	3	x	10

Weight Training

Push-up	4	x	5
DB Push Press	3	x	4
Pull-down	4	x	6
Pull-up	3	x	6

Speed Training

10 yrd Sprint	1	x	10
5-10-5	1	x	5
Speed Ladder	5	x	1

DAY 3

Jump Training

Jump Rope	5	x	25
Jump & Stick	1	x	10
Hop & Stick	2	x	10
Multidirectional	2	x	8
Vertical Jump	3	x	5
Hurdle Jump 28"	3	x	10
Squat Jump	3	x	30

Weight Training

Push-up	3	x	5
DB High Pull	4	x	4
Squat	5	x	6
Step Up (each leg)	3	x	6
DB Bench Press	3	x	6
Pull-down	4	x	6

Speed Training

IS IT FUNCTIONAL?

Gambetta advises that you ask yourself the following questions to determine whether an exercise is, according to a broad, general definition, functional:

Is the movement done in multi-planes?

Is it multi-joint?

Is it high in proprioceptive demand? (Meaning, we have receptors in tendons and joints that we want to challenge.)

The exercise needs to be as fast as we can CONTROL the movement in good form through as great a range of motion.

CHAPTER 8

THE MEDICINE BALL WORKOUT

The first chapter of this book mentions several functional training tools—equipment that can help you to meet your fitness goals in ways that keep your workouts varied and fun. Among the many different pieces of equipment mentioned was the medicine ball, and in this chapter, Paul Frediani, nationally recognized personal trainer, president of Box Athletics and the author of several books on sports specific training, shows you how to do *a complete workout using the ball.*

"The medicine ball is very functional for whatever your sport or fitness goals," says Paul, who frequently uses medicine ball training with his clients. "It increases the intensity of your exercise because your body moves in its own range of motion and is not constrained by a machine." Extremely versatile, the ball can be used for core training, general conditioning and sports-related workouts. Programs designed with the medicine ball effectively work your body in a multi-dimensional way (in three planes of movement), which you'll remember is essential for exercise to be functional and maximally effective.

Like stability balls, medicine balls have been staple weapons in the physical therapy arsenal for decades. They come in a variety of sizes and weights (and colors). You should select a couple of balls of varying weight so that you have a choice depending on the exercise. (Just like you shift between a heavy and light set of dumbbells depending on the exercise.)

Paul finds it amusing when he reads that medicine balls are the hot "new" items in fitness. "Boxers have been using them for years as a means of conditioning," he explains. "They are great to use for anyone who participates in a sport that requires you to stand on your feet and deliver power through your hands by throwing, swinging, rotating, reaching, pulling or pushing. That just about covers **all** sports!"

As an example of the effectiveness of medicine ball training, Paul tells the story of a former Broadway dancer who approached him years ago for boxing lessons: "Roger Puckett was a healthy 57-year-old man who weighed 155 pounds and was in great condition. After he learned the basics in boxing, we started to spar, which is boxing with headgear and larger gloves. While Roger was learning the technique quickly, his movement lacked power. Somewhere between his feet and his hands the power disappeared. So we started a diligent medicine ball workout routine that connected and drove right through his core muscles (the abdominals, hips, and spine). Roger made the mind-body connection and his punches began to have heat in them (I no longer sparred him without my headgear!). He went on to be successful in a couple of boxing matches and is now training for his first bodybuilding competition!"

Pretty impressive stuff. Paul's story points out that no matter how good you may look, or what condition you may think you're in, if you haven't made that core connection you're like the house in the children's story of The Big Bad Wolf: all it will take is a huff and a puff to blow you down. And it should motivate you to pick up a medicine ball the next time you're at the gym, or purchase one for home and try the following complete workout that Paul has designed just for you.

WHAT SIZE MEDICINE BALL IS RIGHT FOR YOU?

Medicine balls come in a variety of weights and diameters. Most commonly they range from 2 pounds to 20 pounds. When choosing a medicine ball select a variety of weights so that you have options depending on the exercise.

PAUL FREDIANI'S MEDICINE BALL WORKOUT

LUNGE SEQUENCE

Perform all lunges by lifting your front foot over an imaginary post that is the height of your knee. The exercises in this series provide full body workouts.

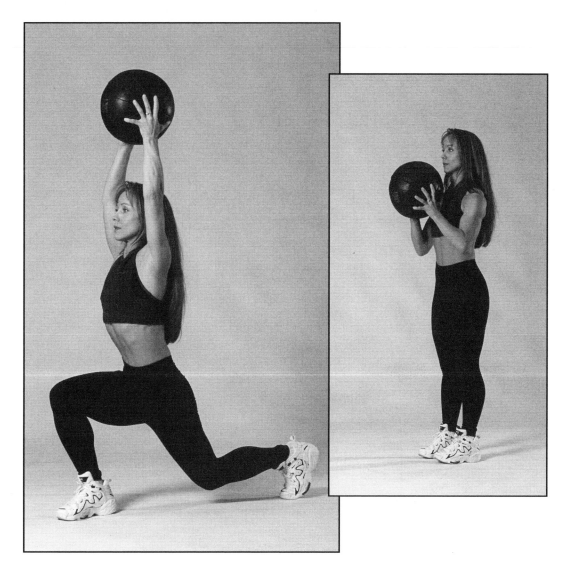

LUNGE PRESS

Hold a medicine ball in your hands. As you lunge forward with one leg press the ball up over your head. Lower the ball as you lunge back to the start position. Switch sides. Do 10-15 times.

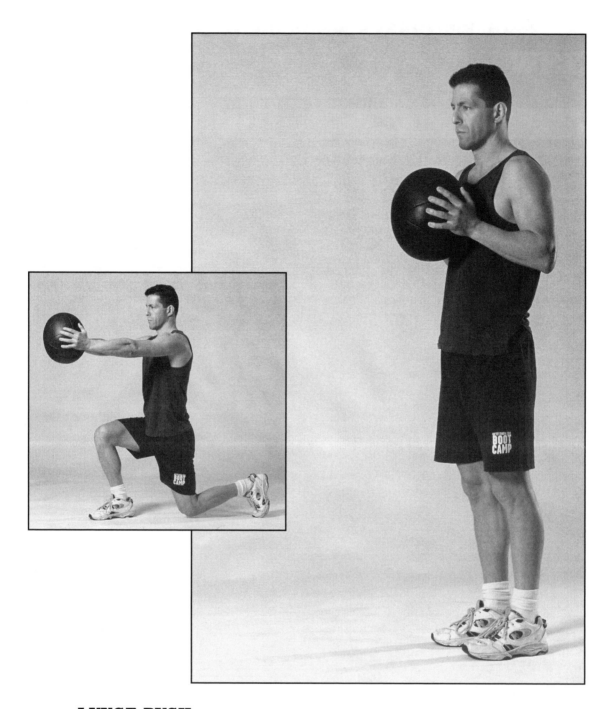

LUNGE PUSH

Hold a medicine ball in your hands. As you lunge forward with one leg push the ball out in front of your chest. Bring it back to your chest as you lunge back to the start position. Switch sides. Do 10-15 times.

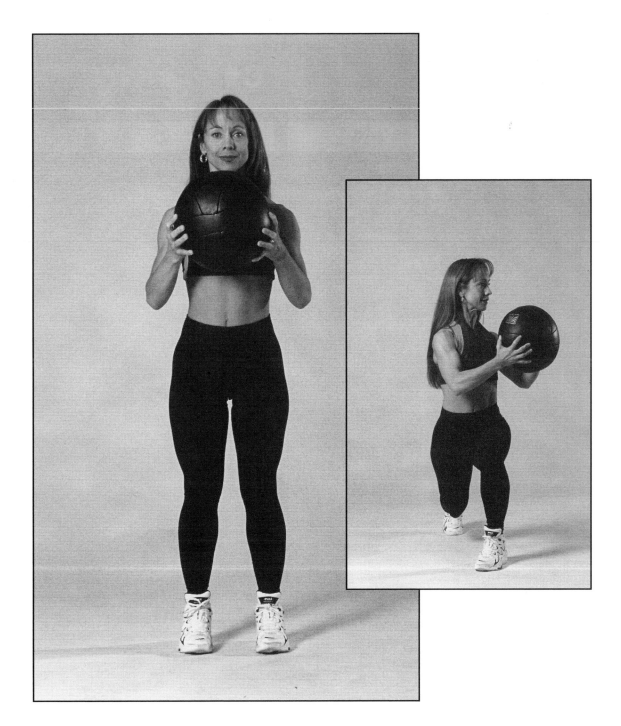

LUNGE TWIST

Hold a medicine ball in your hands. As you lunge forward with your right leg, twist your torso to the right. Return to start position and switch sides. Do 10-15 times on each side.

SQUAT SEQUENCE

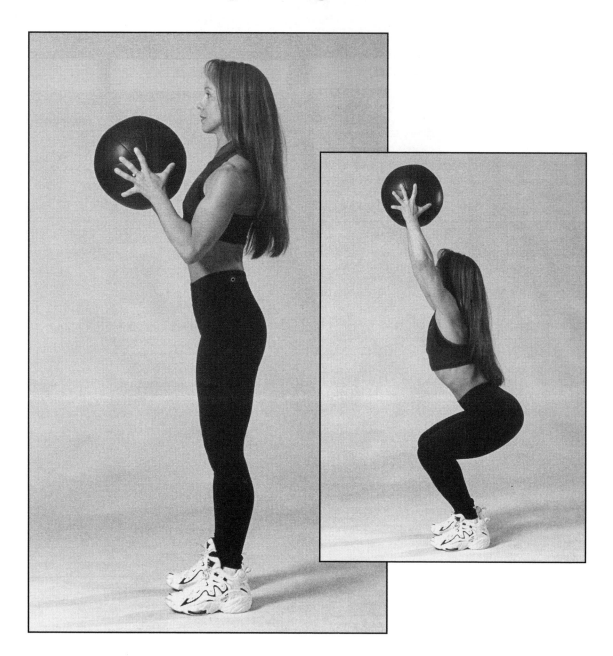

SQUAT PRESS

Hold a medicine ball in your hands. With your feet shoulder width apart, lower your body into a squat position. As you lower, press the ball over your head. Do 10-15 times.

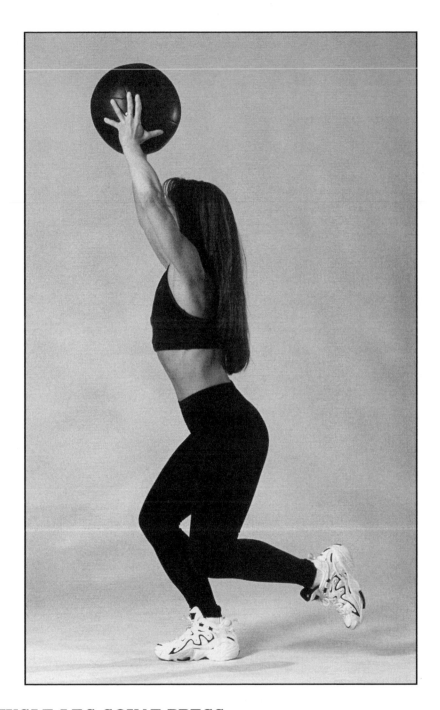

SINGLE LEG SQUAT PRESS

This is the same as the squat press, except you balance on one leg as you go into the squat. Do 10 times on each leg.

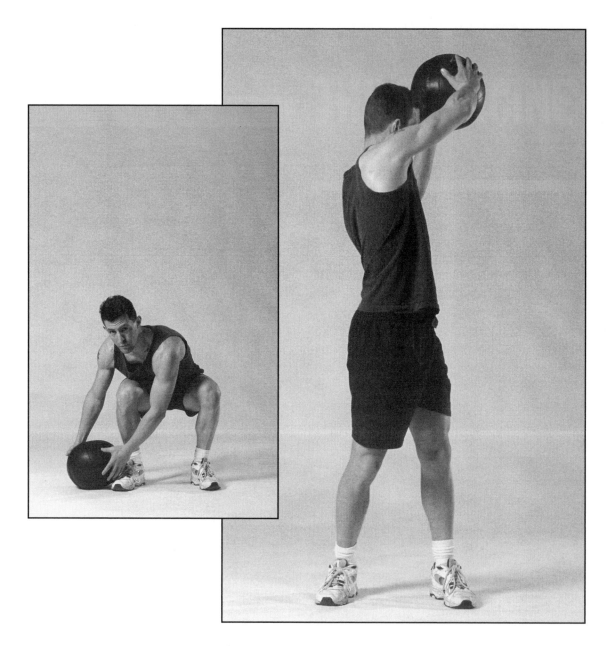

HAYBALERS (KNEE AND ANKLE)
Squat, holding a medicine ball at your right knee then lift the ball across your body over to your left shoulder. Switch sides. Do 10 times on each side. Then, repeat the exercise, beginning this time with the ball next to your right ankle instead of your knee, and lift it over to the opposite shoulder.

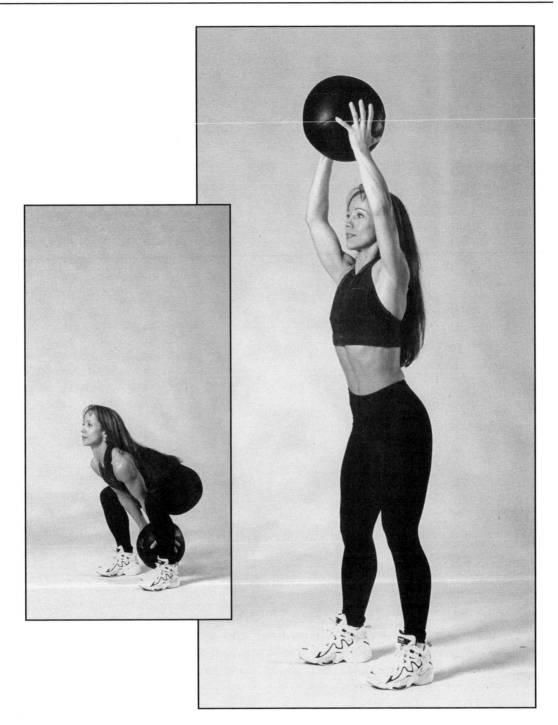

WOOD CHOP

Stand with knees slightly bent, holding the medicine ball over your head. Bend at the waist and push the ball between your legs, then lift back up to overhead position.

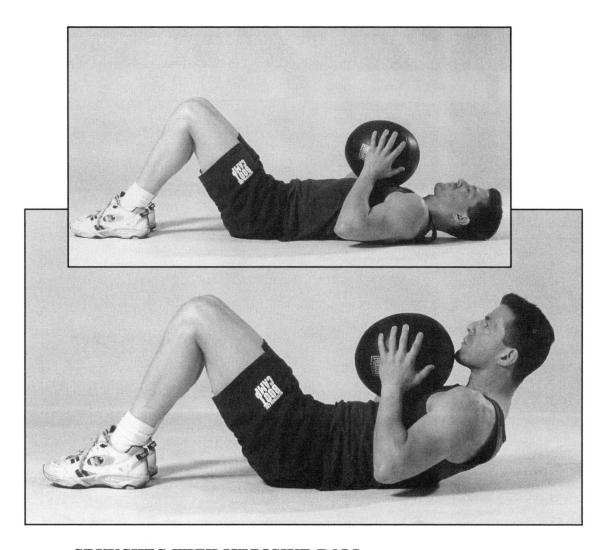

CRUNCHES WITH MEDICINE BALL

Lie on a mat with your knees bent and your lower back pressed against the mat. Holding a medicine ball in your arms, lift your upper body off the mat, then lower back down without letting your shoulders touch the mat.

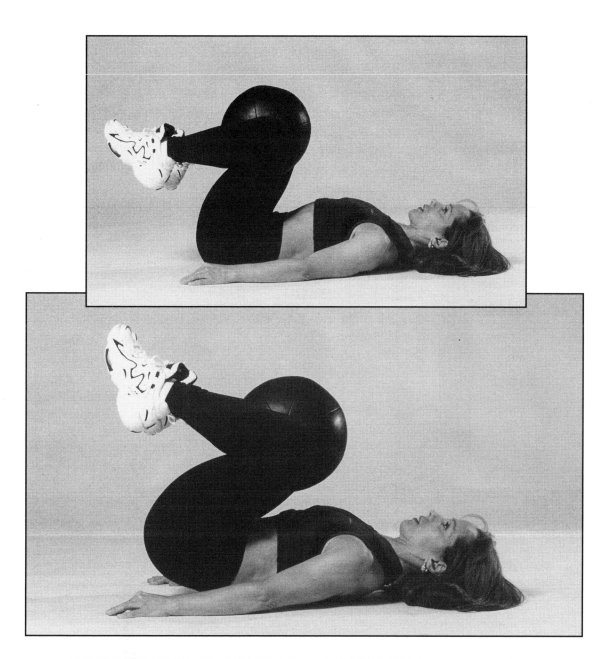

REVERSE SIT-UPS WITH MEDICINE BALL

Lie on a mat with your lower back pressed down. Holding a medicine ball in between your thighs, knees or ankles, bring your knees in toward your chest, lifting your tailbone off the mat. Do 15-20 times. (You can also perform this exercise with your chest lifted).

"Doing the lunge while having the medicine ball tossed to you is one of the most challenging and beneficial exercises I've ever done. It improves my coordination, burns fat and targets every area that I need to strengthen."
—David Weissman, New York, NY

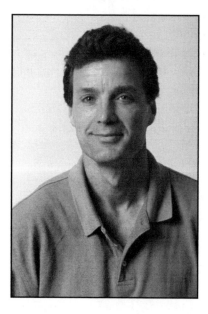

PAUL'S FINAL WORD:

"If you only have three hours a week you can devote to training, then it makes sense to do functional training, such as boot camp classes: they are fun and challenging, and because you keep changing the exercises, you are constantly challenging your neuromuscular system. In short, you get more bang for the buck with functional training."

Paul Frediani, ACSM
President, BoxAthletics
www.paulfrediani.com

CHAPTER 9

CREATING YOUR OWN PROGRAM

Functional training is here to stay. The American Council on Exercise predicts that this new millennium will see a continued increase in both core strength training and exercise classes that are more functional in nature.[1] Now that you've gotten great advice from top experts in the fitness field, it's time to pull the information together so you can create your own functional training program. Remember that each and every one of us is different both physically (we have different shapes, strengths, weaknesses, skills, etc.) and mentally (we all have different goals for ourselves), so the programs must truly be tailored to your particular needs and situation. That said, here's a guide to help you incorporate this exciting type of training into your life!

ASSESS YOUR SITUATION

Before you begin any exercise program, you need to assess your current fitness level. It is only when you know exactly where you are that you can determine where you should go. If you are sedentary and over the age of 30, you should first check with your physician before embarking on any exercise program. It also is a good idea to schedule an appointment with a fitness professional for a health screening and overall fitness assessment. Many health clubs provide such an assessment free to all members. A freelance certified personal trainer will also be able to conduct the assessment. You can locate a certified personal trainer through the American Council on Exercise's webiste at www.acefitness.org., as well as through www.getfitnow.com.

The session should consist of testing in the five categories of fitness: **cardiorespiratory efficiency (your heart/lung fitness), muscular strength, muscular endurance, flexibility and body composition** (how much body fat you have).[2] The goals of the assessment are to assess your current fitness level, to help develop an exercise program, and to identify any health or injury risks. The American College of Sports Medicine recommends that within three hours prior to having your fitness assessment you refrain from eating or drinking alcohol or caffeine; that you come to the assessment well rested (do not exercise right before it—this will throw off results); and that you wear loose fitting clothing that enables you to move freely.3

DETERMINE YOUR GOALS

Once you've completed your assessment and reviewed the results, you and your trainer can determine goals that are appropriate for you. The most important thing to keep in mind is that *your goals need to be realistic.* If you have not done any exercise in the last 10 years and want to become an ace tennis player in three months, you are setting yourself up for disappointment and failure. You didn't get out of shape in three months, you can't expect to get back into shape in three. That doesn't mean you won't see improvements quickly; if you stick to your program you should notice gains in many of the areas of fitness, whether that be better stamina, more strength, etc. within a few weeks. Just be realistic. This is why working with a trainer can be so advantageous; he or she will help to ensure that the goals and resulting program you set up are attainable and bring you success!

When determining your functional training goals, think about the physical things that you currently most enjoy doing or most desire to do in the future. Is it playing football with the kids? Running? Gardening or Carpentry? Rock Climbing? The functional training program that you develop will depend upon your goal. Because your body adapts specifically to exercise, you need to select exercises that reflect the activity that you want to improve in or begin. For example, if you want to ski, you will concentrate on doing exercises that involve your lower body, moving in ways that mimic the stress of skiing. If you want to rock climb, you'll also work on upper body exercises. Of course all of your programs must involve the all-important core conditioning and training exercises that Paul Chek presented in Chapter Four.

DESIGN YOUR PROGRAM

Now that you've had your assessment and determined your goals, ask yourself these questions first presented in Chapter One:

1. What joints are involved in the movement, and how do the muscles work?

2. What is the range of motion at each joint during the activity and exercise?

3. What is the speed of the contraction?

4. What equipment can I use to help to copy the movement?

You and your trainer will develop the appropriate exercises based on your responses to these questions, that will best mimic the desired activity (for example, skiing) and therefore produce that all important transfer of training effect.

As you begin your training program don't forget the general rules for progression:

1. Add resistance gradually.

2. Begin on stable surfaces, progress to unstable ones.

3. Master stability and coordination first.

4. Work on speed and power *only after you have mastered the exercise slowly with control.*

Progressing in a systematic, logical way takes patience—we all tend to want what we want now rather than later; but by working up to your goal you will minimize your risk of injury and maximize your ultimate mastery of the activity.

DON'T FORGET YOUR HEART

The functional training exercises presented in this book are essential to make your body more efficient, stronger and able to accomplish what you want—whether in daily life or on the courts. Many of them—in particular exercises like lunges and squats, will get your heart rate up and may even cause you to sweat. That said, most of them will not give your heart enough of the workout it needs for optimal health and fitness. In other words, you will also need to incorporate aerobic training into your workouts (an exception is a strenuous boot-camp type workout, which typically will keep your heart rate up in what is known as a training zone for most of the class). Technically, aerobic exercises are those that use oxygen in order to produce the cellular energy needed to exert force (called adenosine triphosphate or ATP). Aerobic literally means "with oxygen." These exercises use large muscle groups (namely the legs) and involve sustained movement. Brisk walking, running, swimming, and biking all are examples of aerobic exercise. When you do aerobic exercise, you are bringing oxygen-rich blood to your heart and lungs, and are improving the efficiency of your heart (like giving yourself a heart tune-up)! You should work out aerobically at a level that is challenging, yet achievable (you should be able to talk while running, for example) for 20-60 minutes, at least three days a week.

DEVELOP A WORKABLE SCHEDULE

We're all pressed for time these days. Between work, chores, and family obligations we barely have enough time to eat proper meals, let alone exercise! How can you incorporate a functional training program into your already-tight workout schedule?

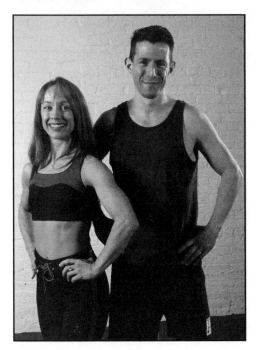

First, determine how much time per week you can devote to your training. BE HONEST HERE! Think about the hours that you may be wasting on Must-See-TV, thumbing through magazines, or not being efficient. All you need to do is to find at least 30 minutes on four days a week to optimize the benefits from your training. Of course, if all you can do is 20 minutes, three days a week, that is still better than nothing and it will do you functional good. But, *if you want to be the best you can be, you'll need to devote more time* (as with everything in life, you need to put the time and effort in to get the reward!)

On the following pages, you will find sample program schedules based on three scenarios: two hours a week, four hours a week and six and a half hours a week. The programs also look at three different levels and overall goals: Program A is for someone who is de-conditioned and wants to improve daily life activities; Program B is for someone of average fitness who wants better overall functional strength and flexibility and Program C is for someone who is already fit and wants to move to the next level in a sport or activity. Each program includes functional training exercises presented in this book as well as schedules for your aerobic exercising. Determine which of these scenarios might work best for you. Or, simply use them as a guide when creating your own program.

THE COMPONENTS OF FITNESS

Contrary to conventional thought, being in shape doesn't solely mean having a well-toned or muscularly developed body. To be truly fit you must have the following:

Muscular Strength: Your muscles must be strong enough to perform all that you need to in life with as much ease as possible.

Muscular Endurance: Your must be able to sustain an activity over time.

Cardiovascular Fitness: Your heart and lungs must be in good working order-achieved through regular aerobic exercise.

Flexibility: You must have ample range of motion around your joints. Take the time to stretch every day!

Body Composition: Your ratio of lean body mass to fat must be in a healthy range.

SAMPLE PROGRAM A

PROFILE: Beginner or deconditioned
GOAL: Improve ability to do daily activities
TIME: Two hours per week

MONDAY:

- 20 minutes of ADL exercises (Chapter Five)
- 10 minutes of stretching (Chapter Three)

WEDNESDAY:

- 20 minutes of aerobic exercise (e.g. brisk walking, jogging or biking)
- 10 minutes of Phase-I core training (Chapter Four)

FRIDAY:

- 15 minutes aerobic exercise
- 10 minutes Phase-I core training (Chapter Four)
- 5 minutes flexibility training (Chapter Three)

SUNDAY:

- 20 minutes of aerobic exercise
- 10 minutes of ADL exercises (Chapter Five)

SAMPLE PROGRAM B

PROFILE: Intermediate or average fitness level
GOAL: Better functional strength
TIME: Four hours per week

MONDAY:

- 30 minutes of aerobic exercise
- 20 minutes of functional strength training
- 10 minutes of core training

WEDNESDAY:

- 30 minutes of aerobic exercise
- 10 minutes of medicine ball training
- 10 minutes of functional strength training
- 10 minutes of flexibility training

FRIDAY:

- 30 minutes aerobic exercise
- 15 minutes core training
- 10 minutes of functional strength training
- 5 minutes of flexibility training

SUNDAY:

- 30 minutes of aerobic exercise
- 20 minutes of medicine ball training
- 10 minutes of core training

SAMPLE PROGRAM C

PROFILE: Advanced or superior fitness level
GOAL: Next level in fitness
TIME: 6.5 hours per week

MONDAY:

- 40 minutes of aerobic exercise
- 20 minutes of functional strength training
- 10 minutes of core training
- 5 minutes of flexibilty training

WEDNESDAY:

- 40 minutes of aerobic exercise
- 20 minutes of sports-specific athletic training
- 10 minutes of flexibility training

THURSDAY:

- 30 minutes aerobic exercise
- 15 minutes core training
- 10 minutes of flexibilty training

FRIDAY:

- 30 minutes aerobic exercise
- 15 minutes core training
- 15 minutes of functional strength training
- 15 minutes of sports-specific athletic training

SUNDAY:

- 45 minutes of aerobic exercise
- 10 minutes of medicine ball training
- 10 minutes of core training
- 20 minutes of sports-specific athletic training
- 5 minutes of flexibilty training

FUNCTIONAL TRAINING

Use these sample schedules as guidelines when creating your own personalized workout plan that is based on your own needs and goals—whether they be related to every day activities, or sports-specific activities. Nothing is written in stone: if you want to spend one day focusing entirely on core training, go ahead. Just be sure that at the end of the week you've struck a reasonable balance in terms of the different types of functional training. Remember, too, that you can supplement your training with fitness classes such as sports conditioning classes, core conditioning classes and boot camp (just be very careful in a group setting of working at the level that's appropriate for you. Never feel compelled to do what everyone else is doing if you are not ready.) Be smart about your training.

FINAL WORDS

Congratulations! Now that you've read this far you can take the information and advice from our noted experts to get you on the road to a more functionally healthy and fit lifestyle. You picked up this book for a reason: perhaps you were intrigued by the title and wondered "what the heck is this about?" Or, perhaps you've been seeing a lot of this type of training and wanted to know how it could possibly fit into your life fitness plan. Well, now you know *and it's entirely up to you to take the next step.* If you do, you will be rewarded with a body that can take you where you want to go; to a place where you will feel more powerful, stronger, and in control. That's a great place to be. So welcome to this exciting new revolution in fitness and, above all, remember to keep the "fun" in functional training!

— RESOURCES —

FUNCTIONAL TRAINING EQUIPMENT—

Get Fit Now Internet Store
www.getfitnow.com
1-800-906-1234

Perform Better
www.performbetter.com
1-800-556-7464

FITNESS NEWS AND EDUCATION—

Personal Training on the Net
www.PtontheNet.com

Get Fit Now Website
www.getfitnow.com

American Council on Exercise
www.acefitness.com

C.H.E.K. Institute
www.chekinstitute.com

Gambetta Sports Training Systems
www.gambetta.com

Perform Enhance
www.performenhance.net

— REFERENCES —

Chapter One:

1. American Council on Exercise. (1997) *Personal Trainer Manual* (1997). San Diego, Ca.: American Council on Exercise. p. 260

2. Stone, Michael H., & Stone, Margaret E. (1998) Training principles *Muscular Development.* Dec., 1998.

3. Cunningham, Christine. (2000). Strengthen clients for everyday activities *Personal Fitness Professional.* April, 2000. p. 22-23.

Chapter Two:

1. Shea, Charles H., Shebilske, Wayne L., & Worchel, Stephen. (1993). Chapter 2: Biological Foundations. (*In Motor Learning and Control*). Upper Saddle River, NJ: Prentice Hall.

2. Chek, Paul. (1999) *The Golf Biomechanics Manual.* Encinatas, CA: C.H.E.K. Institute.

3. Stone, Michael H, & Stone, Margaret E. (1998) Training principles. *Muscular Development.* Dec., 1998.

4. Cunningham, Christine. (2000). Strengthen clients for everyday activities. *Personal Fitness Professional.* April, 2000.

Chapter Three:

4. Borg, G.V. (1982). Psychological basis of perceived exertion. *Medicine and Science in Sports and Exercise.* 14, p. 377-381.

Chapter Four:

1. Chek, Paul. (2000). What is functional exercise? Available at www.personaltraining.com.au.

2. Peter H. (2000). Back to the Basics. *ACSM'S Health & Fitness Journal.* 4 (4), p. 19-25

Chapter Six:

1. Lazowki, D.A., Ecclestone, N,A., Myers, A.M., et al. (1999). A randomized outcome evaluation of group exercise programs in long-term care institutions. *Journal of Gerontology and Biological Medical Sciences.* 54 (12), p. 621-628.

2. Brill, P.A., Probst, J.C., Greenhouse, D.L. (1998). Clinical feasibility of a free-weight strength-training program for older adults. *Journal of American Family Practice.* 11(6), p. 445-451.

3. Santana, Juan Carlos. (2000). Improving quality of life for older adults. *Personal Fitness Professional.* Aug., 2000, p. 22-25.

Chapter Nine:

1. American Council on Exercise News Release. (2000). *American Council on Exercise Makes Fitness Trend Predictions for 2001. New Release: October 11, 2000.* Available at: http://www.acefitness.org/media/media_list_bymonth.cfm

2. American Council on Exercise. (1997) Chapter 6: Testing and Evaluation, p. 169-205. *Personal Trainer Manual.* San Diego, Ca.: American Council on Exercise.

3. American College of Sports Medicine. (2000) *Guidelines for Exercise Testing and Prescription.* 6th Ed. Philadelphia, PA: Lippincott Williams & Wilkins, Philadelphia, p. 52.

— ABOUT THE AUTHOR —

RoseMarie Gionta Alfieri is a certified exercise instructor for The New York Health and Racquet Club in New York City and a freelance writer. RoseMarie has a bachelor's degree in communications from Boston College and a master's degree in health education from Columbia University. She is the author of several articles in the health, fitness and education fields. RoseMarie, who grew up on Long Island and has lived in Manhattan, currently resides in Larchmont, New York.

Here are a few new titles from
Hatherleigh Press/Getfitnow.com Books.

These exciting fitness books are available at your local bookstore or library,
or by ordering direct from the publisher:

TOLL FREE 1-800-906-1234
WEBSITE: GETFITNOW.COM

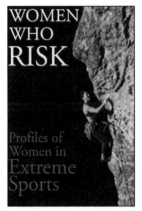

1-57826-092-2 $22.95

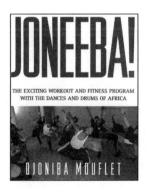

1-57826-049-3 $19.95

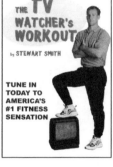

1-57826-020-5 $14.95

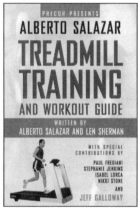

1-57826-080-9 $14.95

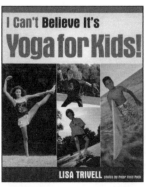

1-57826-044-2 $16.95

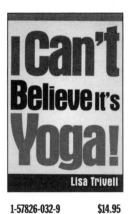

1-57826-032-9 $14.95

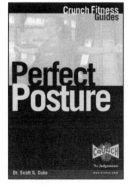

1-57826-040-X $14.95

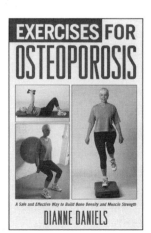

1-57826-076-0 $14.95

Here are a few new titles from
Hatherleigh Press/Getfitnow.com Books.

These exciting fitness books are available at your local bookstore or library,
or by ordering direct from the publisher:

TOLL FREE 1-800-906-1234
WEBSITE: GETFITNOW.COM

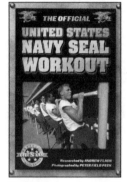

1-57826-009-4 $14.95

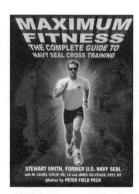

1-57826-060-4 $16.95

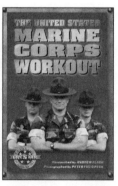

1-57826-011-6 $14.95

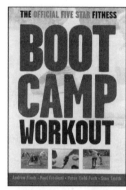

1-57826-033-7 $14.95

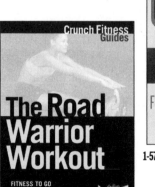

1-57826-025-6 $14.95

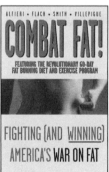

1-57826-089-2 $23.95

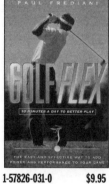

1-57826-031-0 $9.95

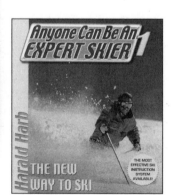

1-57826-073-6 $19.95